T0176468

Migration-sensitive Cancer Registration in Europe

Challenges in Public Health

Editor: Prof. Dr. Oliver Razum, Bielefeld

Formerly/früher: Medizin in Entwicklungsländern
Herausgegeben von
Prof. Dr. Hans Jochen Diesfeld, Heidelberg

Band 62

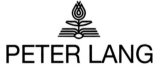

PETER LANG

Frankfurt am Main · Berlin · Bern · Bruxelles · New York · Oxford · Wien

Oliver Razum
Jacob Spallek
Anna Reeske
Melina Arnold
(eds.)

Migration-sensitive Cancer Registration in Europe

Challenges and Potentials

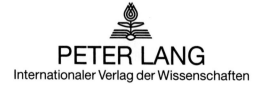

PETER LANG
Internationaler Verlag der Wissenschaften

Bibliographic Information published by the Deutsche Nationalbibliothek
The Deutsche Nationalbibliothek lists this publication in the Deutsche Nationalbibliografie; detailed bibliographic data is available in the internet at http://dnb.d-nb.de.

Cover design: Atelier Platen

The editors' work has partly been funded
under the framework of the Public Health
Programme 2003–2008 of the European Commission
(MEHO project: Migrant and Ethnic Health Observatory;
Contract number: 2005122). The funding agency
had no role in the preparation of the manuscript
or the decision to publish. This work represents
the views of the authors and not necessarily
those of the European Commission.

ISSN 1863-768X
ISBN 978-3-631-61934-6

© Peter Lang GmbH
Internationaler Verlag der Wissenschaften
Frankfurt am Main 2011
All rights reserved.

www.peterlang.de

Foreword

Jan Willem Coebergh

Learning from variation

The EU is a fantastic, peaceful socio-economic challenge. If anything, Europe is about variation, unity in diversity. This becomes also clear when one examines incidence of any disease, certainly also the various cancers: there are always gradients in frequency from north to south and from east to west, also within countries, even the smaller ones. And also in survival being the result of awareness, organization and economic conditions. The gradients also hide ethnic and climatologic variation and of course life style which may largely boil down in socio-economic-cultural differentiation.

If the lowest incidence rates for the various cancers would be attainable across Europe (might still take 50 years or more) then according to a study of Soerjomataram et al. [1] conducted for the Eurocadet FP6 project, the degree of avoidability would be about 40 to 70% of cancers in males and 20 to 50% in females. If there is a negative message from this variation in certain countries, the positive message is that improvement is possible for countries with high incidence, especially also with high mortality rates. But the challenge is also for countries with low incidence rates to avoid deterioration, being also possible, the modern temptations of fast food, alcohol, smoking, quick UV-exposures and mechanization being constantly present. The challenge of not keeping age-at first birth low is of course an intriguing one for women (and men) in most countries being linked to so many competing challenges and opportunities.

Interestingly, in all these domains we can learn a lot from 'our' immigrants, whether they came to seek refuge, economic challenges, love or both. Except for infection-related cancers incidence rates in the countries of origin are usually up to 50% lower, especially for the frequent cancers (in Europe) of the lung, prostate, breast and colorectum. Although their adaptation to the various national cultures and lifestyles is logically strongly stimulated, there is also some logic for the reverse.

This book is certainly shedding further light to this variation and delineate the challenges ahead. Without developing (and implementing) scenarios for cancer prevention many battles for prevention will be lost.

This also makes us realize that we only know much more of all this thanks to the unique network of population-based cancer registries across the EU, each of them also rooted in the variety of medical cultures.

The value of this book is that, for the first time, a broad overview is given on the current situation of migration-sensitive cancer registration in Europe. The barriers but also potentials of this field are being pointed out in a comprehensive way, including evidence from several countries. This work thus serves as a strong basis and guide for prospective cancer registration, monitoring and research lived up to a unified, diverse European society.

The editors of this book are therefore to be complimented with all their work in bringing this together.

Jan Willem Coebergh, MD PhD

Professor of Cancer Surveillance, Erasmus MC Rotterdam, Dept of Public Health

Research-director at Comprehensive Cancer Centre South (IKZ), Eindhoven Cancer Registry

Coordinator of the EU Eurocadet (FP6) and Eurocourse (FP7) projects

References

1. Soerjomataram, I., et al., Excess of cancers in Europe: a study of eleven major cancers amenable to lifestyle change. Int J Cancer, 2007. 120(6): p. 1336-43.

Table of Contents

Table of Contents 9

List of Tables

12   Table of Contents

List of Figures

List of Abbreviations

ANCR	Association of the Nordic Cancer Registries
BKRG	*Bundeskrebsregistergesetz* (Federal Law for Cancer Registries)
BSN	*Burgerservicenummer* (Citizen Service Number)
CBS	Centraal Bureau voor de Statistiek (Statistics Netherlands)
CCC	Comprehensive Cancer Centers
CHI	Community Health Index
CI	Confidence Interval
CSN	Citizen Service Number
DCO	Death Certificate Only
EBV	Epstein-Barr Virus
ECHI	European Community Health Indicators
ECHIM	European Community Health Indicators and Monitoring
ECO	European Cancer Observatory
ENCR	European Network of Cancer Registries
EU	European Union
EUROCHIP	European Cancer Health Indicator Project
FCR	Finnish Cancer Registry
FI	Finland
GDR	German Democratic Republic
GEKID	Association of Population-based Cancer Registries in Germany
GKV	*Gesetzliche Krankenversicherung* (Statutory Health Insurance)
GP	General Practitioner
GPD	Gross Domestic Product
GRELL	*Groupe pour l'Épidémiologie et l'Enregistrement du Cancer dans les Pays de Langue latine* (Group for Cancer Epidemiology and Registration)
GROS	General Register Office for Scotland
HCQI	Health Care Quality Indicators
HPV	Human Papilloma Virus
HSL	*Hälso- och sjukvårdslagen* (Health and Medical Service Act)
IACR	International Association of Cancer Registries
IARC	International Agency for Research on Cancer
ICD	International Classification of Diseases
IKZ	Comprehensive Cancer Center South, Eindhoven Cancer Registry
ISD	Information Services Division
KIGGS	Child and Youth Health Survey
KRG	*Krebsregistergesetz* (Law for cancer registration)
LISA	Longitudinal Integration Database for Health Insurance and Labour Market studies
MBR	Medical Birth Register
MEHO	Migrant and Ethnic Health Observatory
MRR	Mortality Rate Ratios
NCR	Netherlands Cancer Registry
NHI	National Health Insurance
NHS	National Health Service
NL	The Netherlands
OECD	Organisation for Economic Co-operation and Development
PCIR	Proportional Cancer Incidence Ratio
PID	Personal Identity Code

PIN   Personal Identification Number
PKV   *Private Krankenversicherung* (Private Health Insurance)
RIKS-HIA   Register of information and knowledge about Swedish Intensive Heart Care
            admissions
RR   Relative Risk
RSR   Relative Survival Rate
SALAR   Swedish Association of Local Authorities and Regions
SCAAR   Swedish Coronary Angiography and Angioplasty register
SCR   Scottish Cancer Registry
SEP   Socio-economic position
SES   Socio-economic status
SIR   Standardized Incidence Ratio
SMR   Standardized Mortality Ratio
SMR-01   Scottish Morbidity Record
TCR   Tehran Cancer Registry
TNM   Classification of Malignant Tumors (tumor, lymph nodes, metastasis)
UK   United Kingdom
USA   United States of America
UV   Ultraviolet
WHO   World Health Organization

Chapter 1:

Introduction

1. Introduction

Anna Reeske[1], Jacob Spallek[1,2], Melina Arnold[2], Oliver Razum[2]

1 University of Bremen, Bremen Institute for Prevention Research and Social Medicine, Germany
2 Bielefeld University, Department for Epidemiology and International Public Health, Germany

Establishing migration-sensitive cancer registration in Europe would mean establishing a routine monitoring of cancer occurrence in migrant and ethnic minority groups within and between European countries. It is a basic requirement for describing their health status and revealing cancer risk disparities, both between similar migrant groups in different European countries, as well as between migrants and autochthonous populations, in order to develop adequate strategies to prevent or reduce health inequalities between migrants and non-migrants.

The majority of European countries has to face a growing diversity of its populations especially due to heterogeneous groups migrating to Europe or staying there in the second or third generation. Migrants in Europe are quite heterogeneous with respect to origin, age, socioeconomic status, reason of migration, migrant generation as well as health risks and resources. So far, in many European countries, there is a lack of information and data that are collected on these groups. Data are not collected routinely or systematically and hence these countries are not able to obtain an overview of the health situation of the migrants residing there.

Aim of this book is to (i) describe the status quo of migrant-sensitive cancer registration in Europe and (ii) reveal and discuss the potentials regarding a routine monitoring of the health and cancer patterns among migrant populations in Europe. The book will give an overview and methodological discussion of migration-sensitive cancer registration and explain the idea of developing common indicators in order to conduct scientific, potentially transnational, analyses and to perpetuate adequate monitoring of the health of migrant populations in future.

One of the basic problems regarding the lack of health reporting in migrant groups in Europe is the difficulty of defining migrants or ethnic groups. There is no standardised definition available in most EU countries and comparisons between countries are hardly possible. Migration background or ethnicity are often described by approximating measures, e.g. by country of birth, language or origin [1]. In some countries, nationality is the only indicator for migration background. Before it will be possible to monitor and describe cancer patterns (and other health risks and outcomes) among migrants across countries, it has to be agreed on a uniform migrant definition.

In this book, we used a broad definition of 'who is a migrant' in order to take account of the huge number of existing migrant definitions in Europe and to avoid the inclusion of migrants solely based on country of birth or nationality. Furthermore, ethnic minority groups which are not defined as migrants by the common definition are included, when they present an important group in terms of cancer risk patterns (e.g. the Skolts in Finland, see Chapter 4).

Developing migration-sensitive health indicators for monitoring constitutes one of the major aims of the EU-funded Migrant and Ethnic Health Observatory" (MEHO)-project. Some of the results presented in this book are part of MEHO, funded by the European Commission and conducted between 2006 and 2009. The coordination of the project was headed by the Erasmus Medical Center at Rotterdam University. The project comprised nine work packages with associated partners in other European countries[1] and focussed on the lack of routinely collected information on migrant status in health databases and encouraged the EU member states to share experiences regarding this topic.

The main objectives of the MEHO project were
(1) to make an inventory of existing data sources on migrant health across Europe,
(2) to tackle conceptual, methodological, ethical and practical issues of identifying immigrants in these health databases and
(3) to develop recommendations on migrant and ethnic-specific indicators to routinely monitor the health status of migrant groups in six different areas, including cancer and on how to achieve comparability between data bases in the EU countries.

---

1   Partners were:
–   Institute of Health Policy and Management, Erasmus Medical Centre, University Medical Center, Rotterdam, The Netherlands
–   Department of Public Health, Erasmus Medical Centre, University Medical Center, Rotterdam, The Netherlands
–   Lazio Sanità, Agency for Public Health, Rome, Italy
–   Division of Community Health Sciences – Public Health Sciences Section, University of Edinburgh Medical School, Edinburgh, Scotland
–   Faculty of Health Sciences – Institute of Public Health – Department of Health Services Øster, University of Copenhagen, Denmark
–   Economic Department, Institute of Hygiene, University of P.J. Safarik Kosice, Slovakia
–   Department of Public Health Medicine, University of Bielefeld, Germany
–   Faculty for Life Sciences, Hamburg University of Applied Sciences, Germany
–   Department of Epidemiology and International Public Health, School of Public Health, University of Bielefeld, Germany

Cancer was one of the main areas addressed in the MEHO project. Monitoring cancer mortality and incidence among migrants is of particular interest, because studies have shown that cancer risk (for specific cancer sites) can differ between migrants and autochthonous populations [2-5].

During the course of the MEHO project, the Department of Epidemiology & International Public Health at Bielefeld University (Germany) was in charge of the work package "cancer/cancer registration".

Specific objectives of this work package cancer and cancer registration were:

- to identify existing databases in European cancer registries with information on cancer cases/incidence according to migrant status,
- to identify the different ways in which information on migrant status is collected in European cancer registries,
- to assess data on the coverage and completeness of the registries,
- to develop indicators for cancer patterns among immigrants in Europe,
- to develop recommendations for a uniform definition of migrant status in EU cancer registrations and for further improvements of "migrant sensitivity".

Findings of the MEHO project and additional evidence collected emphasise the need for intensified monitoring of cancer risk among migrants. Migration-sensitive cancer research and monitoring have important implications for equity-related health policies and can help to investigate cancer causes. Thus, a functioning network and collaboration of experts in this field is vital and worthwhile.

The first content chapter of the book (chapter 2) depicts a brief outline of the development of cancer registration in Europe. Essential aspects being discussed are the quality, comparability and completeness of data throughout European registries. Against this backdrop, a short introduction on possibilities and difficulties of cancer registry-based migrant research is given.

Chapter 3 addresses theoretical and methodological issues, discussing challenges with respect to definitional difficulties and indicator development in the field of migrants and cancer. Aiming at getting an overview on the current evidence concerning cancer patterns in migrants, a background chapter covers current knowledge of cancer risk diversity in non-Western migrants coming to Europe in comparison to autochthonous populations in Europe based on a literature overview (chapter 3.1). During the MEHO, project the development of indicators was initiated with identifying and compiling the ways information on migrant status is collected in migration-sensitive cancer databases in Europe. Therefore, a survey among all population-based cancer registries in EU-countries was conducted regarding migration-sensitive data collection, coverage and completeness of data. Results of this survey are presented in chapter 3.2.

Based on current literature, survey results and available migration-sensitive health reports, recommendations for a set of indicators, definitions and measures are developed that could be used in migration-sensitive cancer registration and research (chapter 3.3).

The core of the book is constituted by country reports, describing the potentials and barriers concerning migration-sensitive cancer registration and research in these European countries. Case studies of six countries (namely Scotland, Sweden, Finland, Germany, Denmark and The Netherlands) are presented, each arisen from close collaborations with local experts. Every country report contains a description of the specific situation with regard to cancer registration, studies on cancer among migrant populations in this country and possibilities of establishing a routine monitoring or conducting dedicated studies on the cancer risks of migrants (chapter 4).

Finally, the country-specific insights will be summarized, compared and evaluated based on the standards developed in order to provide references for the future (chapter 5).

The editors want to thank all persons involved in compiling this book. We are especially grateful to the (co-)authors of the introducing chapter on cancer registration in Europe as well as the country reports for their valuable and constructive work in writing and approving the chapters.

References

1. Bhopal, R., Glossary of terms relating to ethnicity and race: for reflection and debate. J Epidemiol Community Health, 2004. 58(6): p. 441-5.
2. Hemminki, K., X.J. Li, and K. Czene, Cancer risks in first-generation immigrants to Sweden. International Journal of Cancer, 2002. 99(2): p. 218-228.
3. Spallek, J., et al., Cancer incidence rate ratios of Turkish immigrants in Hamburg, Germany: A registry based study. Cancer epidemiology, 2009. 33(6): p. 413-8.
4. Visser, O. and F.E. van Leeuwen, Cancer risk in first generation migrants in North-Holland/Flevoland, The Netherlands, 1995-2004. Eur J Cancer, 2007. 43(5): p. 901-8.
5. Zeeb, H., et al., Transition in cancer patterns among Turks residing in Germany. Eur J Cancer, 2002. 38(5): p. 705-11.

Chapter 2:

Cancer registration in Europe

2. Cancer registration in Europe

Eva Steliarova-Foucher[1], Max Parkin[2]

1 European Network of Cancer Registries (ENCR), International Agency for Research on Cancer (IARC), Lyon, France.
2 Cancer Research UK, Centre for Epidemiology, Mathematics and Statistics, Wolfson Institute of Preventive Medicine, London, United Kingdom.

2.1 The European Network of Cancer Registries (ENCR)

In Europe, cancer registration has been developing since early 1900s, with a cancer registry starting in 1929 in Hamburg and in 1942 in Denmark. The growing number of cancer registries since 1950s is illustrated in figure 2.1. Currently, cancer registries cover the national populations in 21 European countries, either as a single national registry (Austria, Belarus, Belgium, Bulgaria, Croatia, the Czech Republic, Denmark, Estonia, Finland, Iceland, Ireland, Latvia, Lithuania, Malta, Norway, Russia, Slovakia, Slovenia and Sweden, Ukraine) or through a number of regional registries (Germany, the Netherlands, Portugal, Sweden and the United Kingdom). In other countries, cancer registries cover varying numbers of administrative units; these regional cancer registries cover various percentages of the national population in France, Italy, Poland, Romania, Russia, Serbia, Spain, Switzerland and Turkey. Specialised cancer registries focus on the registration of specific tumour types, such as gynecological, digestive, thyroid, etc. Paediatric cancer registries collect data on cancers occurring in children and sometimes also in adolescents. A map illustrates the current coverage of European population by general population-based cancer registries in figure 2.2.

Fig. 2.1: *Number of population-based registries in Europe in the years shown*

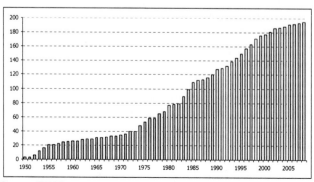

Source: ENCR.

Fig. 2.2:   *Cancer registration coverage in Europe 2010 (source: ENCR)*

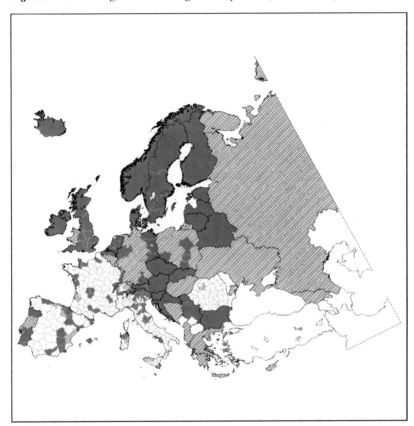

Dark shaded areas refer to registries that were included in at least one of the two most recent volumes of Cancer Incidence in Five Continents.
Hatched areas refer to current/new registries that were not included in the two most recent volumes of Cancer Incidence in Five Continents.

The European Network of Cancer Registries (ENCR) was established in 1989, as a project co-funded by the Europe against Cancer Programme of the European Commission and the International Agency for Research on Cancer (IARC). Since then, the ENCR evolved in an ever-growing network. The aim of the ENCR is to promote collaboration between cancer registries and improve quality and availability of cancer data in Europe.

The ENCR is directed by a Steering Committee, composed of elected, nominated and co-opted members, each staying on the committee for a limited period of time. The nominated members represent the International Agency for

Research on Cancer (IARC), the International Association of Cancer Registries (IACR), the Association of the Nordic Cancer Registries (ANCR) and the *Groupe pour l'Épidémiologie et l'Enregistrement du Cancer dans les Pays de Langue latine* (GRELL). The other five or more members of the committee are elected by the ENCR membership. The members of the network are all population-based cancer registries or their networks operating in Europe. Currently, ENCR has almost 200 members.

Since its inception, the IARC has provided a secretariat to the ENCR. The role of the secretariat includes raising funds to cover the core activities of the Network, organizing meetings, ensuring communication within and outside the network and contributing to all other activities. Most importantly, IARC assembles and disseminates the European cancer data. The secretariat also maintains the ENCR web-site, which provides further information about the network.

2.2 Achieving high data quality and comparability throughout Europe

In almost all European countries, cancer registration is regulated by law[2]. The laws aim at ensuring registration of all new cancer cases and its procedures, especially with respect to protection and confidentiality of personal data. Depending on the laws and the extent of their enforcement, registration practices vary from country to country. In consequence, data quality as well as completeness of ascertainment may be affected by the legal requirements. For example, the impossibility of linking the registered cancer cases with the national (or regional) database of all causes of death (based on identifiable individuals) compromises completeness of registration and a convenient method of long-term follow-up is unavailable. Linkage of the cancer registry database with other national databases greatly increases the quality and value of data collected in all of the linked databases. Cohort studies can be set up to study an association of risk factors and disease on a large scale and aetiological hypotheses may be formulated.

Apart from legal regulations, international comparability of results is also affected by the differences in cancer registration practices and techniques adopted by the individual cancer registries. In order to limit their impact, ENCR mandated several working groups to develop recommendations for collection and coding of various data items, such as definition of date of incidence, coding of most valid basis of diagnosis, method of cancer detection in relation to screening, and others [1]. Registries choose to follow these recommendations in order to foster their participation in international studies, such as CI5 [2].

---

2   Responses to the ENCR Questionnaire 2010 (unpublished data).

ENCR also organises courses for cancer registries personnel to teach best practice in cancer registration and methods of data analysis. Structured registry reviews represent a complementary activity, whereby a single registry is visited by a team of peers, to formally review the registration process, assess its qualities and shortcomings and issue recommendations for further comprehensive development of the registry. Finally, ENCR scientific meetings are organized every few years to permit knowledge exchange amongst the network members.

Participation in international studies further improves data comparability. In the past, the assembled data were stored and distributed to the contributors within the "EUROCIM" software [3]. Although this allowed rather advanced data analysis, there were no criteria of data quality limiting contributions to the database, which made interpretation of results problematic. Currently, a peer review process is being developed with a financial support by the European Commission, to facilitate interpretation of the results.

2.3 Completeness of cancer registration in Europe

The primary concern of all cancer registries is to register all cancer cases newly occurring in the residents of a defined geographical area over a specified time period. By its conception, a population-based cancer registry is the most complete source of data on new cancer cases in a given population. A number of methods are used to measure completeness of cancer registration [4]. Semi-quantitative methods give an indication of the degree of completeness relative to other data sets (within the same registry, in other registries or over time). Quantitative techniques provide a numerical evaluation of the extent to which all eligible cases have been registered, based on assumptions about data flow and assessment of the proportionate representation of the possible data sources among the registered cases. Some of these methods are relatively new and can only be used in those cancer registries where required non-standard variables are collected. For example, to use 'flow method' [5], a registry needs to collect variables 'date of registration' and 'first notified from a death certificate' and has to follow-up all registered cases for vital status. Repeated specific studies are necessary to monitor completeness over time on a regular basis. The majority of cancer registries have assessed formally completeness of their registries in ad-hoc studies [6]. In the peer reviewed international comparative incidence studies [2, 7] the completeness has been routinely assessed by semi-quantitative methods. These methods currently provide the best possible solution for verification of data comparability in a collaborative study of many participating registries.

2.4 Networking on a European basis: Future potentials

Over a period of 2009-2012, ENCR is conducting a major project entitled EUROCOURSE (EUROpe against Cancer: Optimisation of the Use of Registries for Scientific Excellence). The main purpose of EUROCOURSE is to improve the use of cancer registries in European countries through program owners' and researchers' networking, information exchange and benchmarking of best practice. EUROCOURSE is funded within the 7th Framework Programme of the Directorate General Research of the European Commission as an ERA-NET project and it is presented in more detail at its web-site.

EUROCOURSE permits intense networking of ENCR members and other stakeholders, with the aim of promoting modern design of centralised systems of data collection, management, quality control, analysis, presentation, sharing, dissemination and protection. In addition, the role of population-based cancer registries is also being explored in the boundary areas of cancer screening, bio-banking and clinical care. The aim is to render the precious data collected in the cancer registries as useful as possible in all relevant areas of public health and research.

European cancer registries publish data that are used to produce national estimates of cancer incidence (for the countries not covered by a national cancer registry) and allow thus international comparisons. Such estimates have been produced and distributed with specialized software EUCAN [8]. More recently, up-to-date estimates are made available at the web-site of the European Cancer Observatory (ECO). A range of the national estimates of cancer incidence and mortality is illustrated in Fig. 2.3 [9].

2.5 Registry-based research on migrants

Migrant studies provide a useful insight into the relative importance of environment and genetic make-up in disease aetiology. Disease risk is compared between populations of similar genetic background living in different physical and social environments. Migrant studies imply that the groups studied have moved to their new environment relatively recently, and their disease risk can be compared not only with that of the indigenous (host) population, but also with that in their place of origin. Studies of migrants may be differentiated from studies of sections of population based on racial, ethnic, language and religious criteria, although the basic objective of distinguishing the external from internal risk factors may be similar. With respect to the variable "ethnicity", studies within multi-ethnic societies living in a single country are more valuable than between-country comparisons, if the primary variable of interest is ethnicity or racial

Fig. 2.3:   *Estimated incidence and mortality from All sites but non-melanoma skin cancer in the European countries, 2008. The bars represent the Age Standardised Rate (European standard) per 100,000 inhabitants*

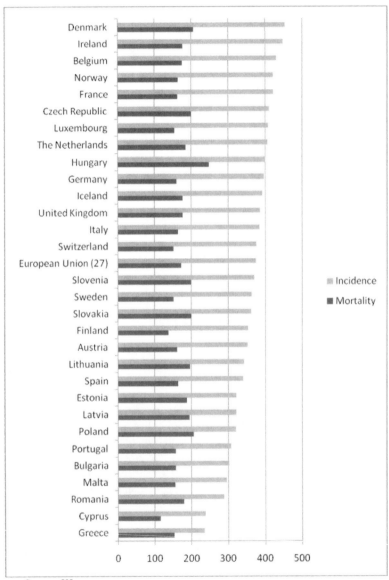

group, since the environmental and social background is likely to be more comparable within a single country than between several countries.

The most common classification of migrant status is by place of birth, a relatively well-defined, unchanging attribute, which is likely to be comparable between the data sources being used (census, vital statistics, cancer registry, etc.). Place of birth can also be used in the study of migrants between neighbouring countries [10-11] or within one country (internal migration) [12-15]. Citizenship or nationality may be recorded by registries [16], although this information is less useful than place of birth, since migrants may become naturalised to varying degrees, and there are more problems of definition (e.g. dual nationality, stateless persons).

Studies that employ a combination of ethnic group and birthplace to distinguish first-generation migrants and their offspring are much more informative than either one alone. The study of disease risk in relation to duration of residence in the new country, or, alternatively, according to the age at the time of migration, is feasible when information is available on the date of migration of the individuals [17-19].

In a survey of cancer registries in the European Union carried out in the late 1990s [20], information about the ethnic group or race was not collected by any of the 69 respondents (out of 95 registries contacted). In the same survey, five registries reported that population data were available by ethnic group or religion. Many registries collected information relevant to the migrant status, such as place of birth (N=41, 51%), country of birth (N=37, 48.1%), year of immigration (N=7, 17%) or religion (N=2, 4.5%). This information may be available to registries through linkage to population registers, in which migrant status (generally country of birth) and date of migration are recorded. In another survey, carried out 15 years later, 78 registries responded out of 191 invited [16]. Among these, country of birth was recorded by 35 (45%) registries, while nationality was recorded in 6 (8%) of the registries and race in only 3 (4%) registries. No migrant-specific data were collected in 44% of those registries.

It is essential that the definition of migrant status is the same in the census and case data, but even with the same definition, individuals may be classified in a different way in the two sources. Lilienfeld and colleagues present unpublished data on differences between country-of-birth statements on death certificates and census returns for the U.S.A. in 1960 – this varied from a 10.8% deficit for U.K. birth to 16.7% excess for Ireland birth on death certificates [21]. The problem is even more acute with respect to ethnicity. In cancer registry data, this variable, if recorded, will be derived from case records, in which determination of ethnicity has most likely been made by health service personnel. In census the ethnicity is usually self-determined and in recent years the individuals are allowed to assign themselves to several ethic groups simultaneously. On European level, statistics with a breakdown by ethnic group or religion are not provided by Eurostat, the statistical office of the EC. In general, ethnic group is a complicated subject (as explained above), and even where statistics are collected it can be misleading to compare data from different countries [22]. However, even if migrant status (or ethnicity) is not available for the population at risk, studies of disease risk are possible using denominator free (proportionate or case control) methodology [23].

In many countries the migrant status in the registered subjects is not routinely recorded and individual linkage of records cannot be performed. Particular methods have been used nevertheless, to address the cancer burden in migrants. In Germany, a name-based algorithm was developed to identify immigrants of Turkish origin [24-25]. Proportional incidence ratios were then used to compare relative occurrence of different cancer types in comparison to the native population [26-27]. A similar technique of name-based algorithms was used to distinguish the UK residents of south Asian origin in studies of the ethnicity and cancer [28-29]. Although the name-based algorithms have apparently high specificity close to 100%, the predictive value is usually poor because of the low prevalence of "ethnics", which results in a lot of misclassification [25]. In addition, this method does not account for loss of the ethnic names through mixed marriages or naturalisation. Another approach may be to obtain ethnicity by linkage to hospital episode statistics [30]. The categorisation of the individuals will depend on question under study: if migrant status is of interest, the country of birth and the date of migration should be available. The study of ethnic group is much more difficult, because many more variables may need to be assessed simultaneously: place of birth, ascendance, nationality, name, phenotype, religion and possibly lifestyle.

Currently, due to the status of data availability, it is not feasible on European level to conduct a study of cancer incidence in migrants to Europe. Standard definitions and procedures, additional resources and possibly also a legislative modifications would be necessary to permit such research.

Nevertheless, it is possible and useful to study cancer burden in migrant populations in specially designed studies as demonstrated above. The differences in cancer incidence risks may inspire research into cancer aetiology. The differences in health care provision should provide impetus for ensuring equity between population subgroups. With the increasing mobility of populations and mixing of cultures worldwide, it may become increasingly difficult to study migrant-specific cancer patterns, which will though tend to fade as this process continues.

Suggested web-based resources

Association of the Nordic Cancer Registries (ANCR): http://www.ancr.nu/
EUROpe against Cancer: Optimisation of the Use of Registries for Scientific Excellence
(EUROCOURSE): http://www.eurocourse.org/
European Cancer Observatory (ECO): http://eu-cancer.iarc.fr/
European Network of Cancer Registries (ENCR): http://www.encr.com.fr/
Groupe pour l'Epidémiologie et l'Enregistrement du Cancer dans les Pays de Langue latine
(GRELL): http://www.grellnet.org/
International Agency for Research on Cancer (IARC): http://www.iarc.fr/
International Association of Cancer Registries (IACR): http://www.iacr.com.fr/

References

1. Standards and Guidelines for Cancer Registration in Europe 2003, in IARC Technical Publication, Tyczynski JE, Demaret E, and Parkin DM, Editors, IARC: Lyon.

2. Cancer incidence in five continents. Volume IX. 2008/01/01 ed. IARC Sci Publ, ed. M.P. Curado, et al. 2008, Lyon. 1-837.

3. ENCR, Eurocim version 4.0. 2001, European Network of Cancer Registries: Lyon.

4. Parkin, D.M. and F. Bray, Evaluation of data quality in the cancer registry: principles and methods Part II. Completeness. European journal of cancer (Oxford, England: 1990), 2009. 45(5): p. 756-64.

5. Bullard, J., et al., Completeness of cancer registration: a new method for routine use. Br J Cancer, 2000. 82(5): p. 1111-6.

6. Schmidtmann, I. and M. Blettner, How Do Cancer Registries in Europe Estimate Completeness of Registration? Methods Inf Med, 2009. 3: p. 267-271.

7. Steliarova-Foucher, E., et al., Quality, comparability and methods of analysis of data on childhood cancer in Europe (1978-1997): report from the Automated Childhood Cancer Information System project. European journal of cancer (Oxford, England: 1990), 2006. 42(13): p. 1915-51.

8. Ferlay, J., et al., EUCAN: Cancer Incidence, Mortality and Prevalence in the European Union 1998. 1999, IARCPress, Lyon.

9. ECO. European Cancer Observatory. [cited 2011 10 Feb]; Available from: http://eu-cancer.iarc.fr.

10. Nilsson, B., et al., Cancer Incidence in Estonian Migrants to Sweden. International Journal of Cancer, 1993. 55(2): p. 190-195.

11. Hemminki, K. and X. Li, Cancer risks in Nordic immigrants and their offspring in Sweden. European journal of cancer (Oxford, England: 1990), 2002. 38(18): p. 2428-34.

12. Borras, J.M., et al., Cervical cancer: incidence and survival in migrants within Spain. J Epidemiol Community Health, 1995. 49(2): p. 153-7.

13. Conti, E.M., et al., Cancer risk related to uncommon migration within Italy. Tumori, 1994. 80(2): p. 101-5.

14. Russo, A., et al., [Incidence of cancer in migrants: data of the Lombardy tumor registry]. Epidemiol Prev, 1994. 18(59): p. 125-32.

15. Rosso, S., et al., Cancer incidence in Turin: the effect of migration. Tumori, 1993. 79(5): p. 304-10.

16. Reeske, A., J. Spallek, and O. Razum, Migrant and Ethnic Health Observatory (MEHO): Migrant-sensitive cancer registration in Europe – Results of a survey conducted among European cancer registries., in Network Eurolifestyle, Neumann G and Kirch W, Editors. 2008, Thieme Verlag: Stuttgart. p. 11-18.

17. Mousavi, S.M., et al., Cancer incidence among Iranian immigrants in Sweden and Iranian residents compared to the native Swedish population. European Journal of Cancer, 2010. 46(3): p. 599-605.

18. Norredam, M., et al., Differences in stage of disease between migrant women and native Danish women diagnosed with cancer: results from a population-based cohort study. Eur J Cancer Prev, 2008. 17(3): p. 185-90.

19. Stirbu, I., et al., Cancer mortality rates among first and second generation migrants in the Netherlands: Convergence toward the rates of the native Dutch population. Int J Cancer, 2006. 119(11): p. 2665-72.

20. Storm, H., I. Clemmensen, and R. Black, Survey of Cancer Registries in the European Union. IARC Technical report 1998. No. 28.

21. Lilienfeld, A.M., M.L. Levin, and I.I. Kessler, Mortality among the foreign born and in their countries of origin, in Cancers in the United States, A.M. Lilienfeld, M.L. Levin, and I.I. Kessler, Editors. 1972, Harvard University Press: Cambridge, Massachusetts. p. 233–278.

22. EUROSTAT. 2010.

23. Kaldor, J., et al., Log-linear models for cancer risk among migrants. Int J Epidemiol, 1990. 19(2): p. 233-9.

24. Spallek, J., et al., [Name-based identification of cases of Turkish origin in the childhood cancer registry in Mainz]. Gesundheitswesen, 2006. 68(10): p. 643-9.

25. Razum, O., H. Zeeb, and S. Akgun, How useful is a name-based algorithm in health research among Turkish migrants in Germany? Tropical medicine & international health: TM & IH, 2001. 6(8): p. 654-61.

26. Spallek, J., et al., Cancer patterns among children of Turkish descent in Germany: a study at the German Childhood Cancer Registry. BMC Public Health, 2008. 8: p. 152.

27. Zeeb, H., et al., Transition in cancer patterns among Turks residing in Germany. Eur J Cancer, 2002. 38(5): p. 705-11.

28. Dos Santos Silva, I., et al., Lifelong vegetarianism and risk of breast cancer: a population-based case-control study among South Asian migrant women living in England. Int J Cancer, 2002. 99(2): p. 238-44.

29. Winter, H., et al., Cancer incidence in the south Asian population of England (1990-92). Br J Cancer, 1999. 79(3-4): p. 645-54.

30. Ali, R., et al., Cancer incidence in British Indians and British whites in Leicester, 2001-2006. Br J Cancer, 2010. 103(1): p. 143-8.

Chapter 3:

Cancer in Migrants

3. Cancer in Migrants

3.1 Cancer in migrant populations: An overview of the literature

Melina Arnold, Oliver Razum

Bielefeld University, Department for Epidemiology and International Public Health, Germany

Migration has become an important phenomenon in Western Europe in terms of population changes, inducing an increasing degree of heterogeneity in European societies during past decades. In 2010, Western and Central Europe host 51 million migrants – defined as foreign born persons – strongly increasing in most recent years. According to the World Migration Report 2010, the majority of migrants to Europe originates from rapidly declining populations, is the result of family reunifications and further due to natural growth of long-term foreign born populations [1]. This development poses major challenges to health care systems and policies, requiring evidence-based research in order to ensure appropriate and individual health care of high quality and effectiveness [2-3].

Migrant populations are exposed to a unique constellation of risk factors that are determined by extrinsic factors and disease patterns experienced in both their country of origin and their host country [4-5]. Cancer, as a multi-causal chronic disease, varies strongly between and within populations as well as geographically, which makes it an ideal setting for studying the impact as well as the interaction of genetic and (abruptly changing) environmental risk factors on carcinogenesis. The comparison of populations of similar genetic background but different environments (migrants vs. country of origin) and of populations of different genetic background but same environment (migrants vs. host country) allows for inferences about aetiology [6]. In this context, the individual life course and particularly early life experiences (as the first step in carcinogenesis) play a major roles in the effects of exposure and their association with cancer risks [7-8].

All-cancer

A generally lower cancer risk in migrants from low-incidence countries has been observed in the majority studies from various European countries, similarly in studies from Australia [9] and the United States [10]. This pattern seems to be due to a retention of favourable risk patterns at the time of migration and thereafter. Changes in cancer risk over time and generation may serve as indications for mainly environmentally mediated causes, responsible for the convergence of rates towards those of the host population respectively. However, there are strong site- and origin-specific differences [11].

Cancer of the lip, oral cavity and pharynx (ICD10: C00-C14)

Risks for cancers of the oral cavity were found to be low in Turkish migrants to Germany [12], North African migrants to the Netherlands [13], West African as well as South East Asian migrants to France [14-15] and Iranian migrants to Sweden [16]. In contrast, studies revealing elevated risks have been conducted in the UK among migrants from South East Asian [17-19] and East African [20] countries. Nasopharyngeal cancer was found to be increased in many studies for migrants of various origin [13-14, 17, 21-22], possibly caused by an infection with the Epstein-Barr virus (EBV).

Cancer of digestive organs (C15-C26)

Favourable risks in migrants were found for oesophageal, colorectal and pancreatic cancers [12-14, 16, 18, 23], whereas risks for cancer of the stomach, liver and gallbladder were often high in migrants [13, 15, 18-19, 23-26], often assumed to be driven by infections caught in early life. In addition, a study from the Netherlands [27] found significant differences between cardia (higher risk in migrants) and non-cardia (lower risk in migrants) stomach cancer, being due to different underlying risk factors.

Cancer of the lung and trachea (C33/34)

The vast majority of studies investigating lung cancer risk in migrant groups, found lower risks compared to the native population of their country of residence. Nevertheless, big gender-specific differences have been observed. In comparison to the population of their host country, females consistently show significantly lower risks, but particularly male migrants from Turkey [12, 28] and Eastern Europe [25, 28] exhibit elevated risks that are very likely to be associated with an increasing and rapid adaptation of smoking patterns in Western countries.

Melanoma (C43/44)

Consistently lower risks for melanoma were confirmed from multiple studies for migrants from various non-Western origins.

Cancer of the breast and female genital organs (C50-C58)

A recent literature review on breast cancer among immigrants [29] revealed favourable (but diverging) risks, pointing towards strong influence of potentially modifiable environmental and behavioural factors and to a lesser degree towards genetic factors. In migrant women, originating from countries with low breast cancer incidences, favourable risks were retained after migration to high incidence countries, although increasing among young migrants and with increasing duration of residence. Breast cancer risks in subsequent generations were observed to be higher than in the first generation migrants. This change in risk over time seems to be caused by acculturation processes and lifestyle modification. One of the main risk factors for breast cancer, age at first birth, seems to play a significant role in carcinogenesis. In a recent study from Sweden [30], early-life exposures were found to contribute significantly to breast cancer risk in later life and suggest the determination of risks before adulthood – and thus, often before migration. This concept explains higher breast cancer risks among migrant women, who migrated at younger ages and among second generation migrants.

The majority of studies on breast cancer in migrants populations reported significantly lower breast cancer risks and mortality in women originating from low income (and often low incidence) countries compared to the native population of their country of residence. This has been confirmed in migrants from Turkey [12-13, 23, 27, 31-32], Eastern Europe [25, 31, 33-34], North Africa [13-14, 34-35], the Middle East [35-36], Asia [17-18, 34, 37-38] and South America [13, 20, 23, 31-32] to Western European countries. In contrast, migrant women from West Africa exhibited significantly elevated risks [20, 34].

Despite equally low risks for cancer of the ovary and the corpus uteri, significantly elevated risks were found for cervical cancer [13, 15, 19-20, 39-40], possibly related to a higher prevalence of HPV infections in less-developed countries.

Cancer of male genital organs (C60-C63)

Migrants from non-Western countries exhibited lower risks for testicular cancer in comparison to the autochthonous population of their country of residence, confirmed by studies conducted in Denmark [41], Sweden [16, 28], the Netherlands [13] and the UK [18, 20]. In contrast, prostate cancer was found to be significantly elevated in West African [20, 34] and South American males residing in the UK [20, 38], although the majority of studies showed lower risks.

Cancer of urinary organs (C64-C68)

Some studies found elevated bladder cancer risks in male migrants from Eastern Europe [31] and the Middle East [16] living in Sweden and West African males residing in France [24]. For the other sites, generally lower risks were observed.

Cancer of the eye, brain and central nervous system (C69-C72)

Low risks for cancer of the brain were revealed in migrants from Turkey [23], African countries [13, 28], South East Asia [15, 18] and South America [13, 20, 23, 28].

Cancer of the thyroid gland (C73)

Increased risks in cancer of the thyroid gland were observed in many studies, for instance in migrants from Turkey [13], North Africa [13], the Middle East [16, 42], South East Asia [18, 21] and in migrants of second generation from Eastern Europe [43]

Hodgkin's disease, lymphoma and leukaemia (C81-C96)

Elevated risks for Hodgkin's disease were found in migrants from Turkey [12-13], South America [13] and in males from South East Asia [18, 21]. Lymphoma were also elevated in Turkish migrants residing in Germany [12, 44], South Asian and South American [20] migrants in the UK [19]. No distinct patterns could be observed for leukaemia.

In summary, there is evidence that migrants from non-Western (and often low incidence) countries were more likely to develop cancers that are related to infectious diseases, compared to the general population of their industrialized host country. This especially holds for cancers of the oral cavity, nasopharynx, stomach, liver, gallbladder, cervix uteri, prostate and lymphomas. In contrast, lower risks were found for cancers that have a strong association with a 'Western' lifestyle (poor diet, physical inactivity, reproductive factors, etc.), such as colorectal cancer and cancers of the pancreas, lung, breast, ovary, kidney and bladder. More conceptually, rates in migrants from low-risk populations increase after migration to high-risk countries. Furthermore, it has been observed that migrants often show cancer risks that are in-between the corresponding risk of the native populations in their home and their host country. However, risks in subsequent generations were observed to further approximate (converge towards) those of the host population [6, 23, 45], pointing towards the concept of acculturation-based health transition [46]. In this context, it has also been shown that migrants from low-incidence countries can also serve as a model for studying risk factors that are suspected to be responsible for rises or differences in cancer risks in high-incidence countries over the course of several decades [30].

Findings from studies on cancer risk in migrant populations may help solving unclear aetiology questions and conducting targeted research in this field.

Furthermore, improved prevention strategies can be derived from migrant studies, being of high value for both migrant populations – in the sense of culturally sensitive prevention – and the majority population – in terms of the disclosure of (new?) risk factors, possibly giving rise to new prevention methods. Given the above facts, the public health relevance and the necessity of migration-specific research is apparent.

Methodological issues for studies investigating cancer occurrence in migrant populations (e.g. bias peculiar to migrant studies and explanatory variables) are discussed in chapter 3.3.

References

1. IOM, World Migration Report 2010. The Future Of Migration: Building Capacities For Change. 2010, International Organization for Migration (IOM): Geneva.
2. Bhopal, R.S., Ethnicity, Race, and Health in Multicultural Societies: Foundations for Better Epidemiology, Public Health, and Health Care. 2007: Oxford Univ Pr.
3. Spallek, J. and O. Razum, [Health of migrants: deficiencies in the field of prevention]. Med Klin (Munich), 2007. 102(6): p. 451-6.
4. Marmot, M., Changing places changing risks: the study of migrants. Public Health Rev, 1993. 21(3-4): p. 185-95.
5. Razum, O. and D. Twardella, Time travel with Oliver Twist--towards an explanation foa a paradoxically low mortality among recent immigrants. Trop Med Int Health, 2002. 7(1): p. 4-10.
6. Parkin, D.M. and M. Khlat, Studies of cancer in migrants: rationale and methodology. Eur J Cancer, 1996. 32A(5): p. 761-71.
7. Zeeb, H., J. Spallek, and O. Razum, [Epidemiological perspectives of migration research: the example of cancer]. Psychother Psychosom Med Psychol, 2008. 58(3-4): p. 130-5.
8. Spallek, J. and O. Razum, Erklärungsmodelle für die gesundheitliche Situation von Migrantinnen und Migranten, in Health Inequalities: Determinanten und Mechanismen gesundheitlicher Ungleichheit U. Bauer, U.H. Bittlingmayer, and M. Richter, Editors. 2008, Vs Verlag: Wiesbaden. p. 271-288.
9. McCredie, M., M.S. Coates, and J.M. Ford, Cancer incidence in migrants to New South Wales. Int J Cancer, 1990. 46(2): p. 228-32.
10. McDonald, J.T. and J. Neily, Race, Immigrant Status, and Cancer Among Women in the United States. J Immigr Minor Health, 2009.
11. Arnold, M., O. Razum, and J.W. Coebergh, Cancer risk diversity in non-western migrants to Europe: An overview of the literature. European journal of cancer (Oxford, England: 1990), 2010. 46(14): p. 2647-59.
12. Spallek, J., et al., Cancer incidence rate ratios of Turkish immigrants in Hamburg, Germany: A registry based study. Cancer epidemiology, 2009. 33(6): p. 413-8.
13. Visser, O. and F.E. van Leeuwen, Cancer risk in first generation migrants in North-Holland/Flevoland, The Netherlands, 1995-2004. Eur J Cancer, 2007. 43(5): p. 901-8.
14. Bouchardy, C., et al., Cancer mortality among north African migrants in France. Int J Epidemiol, 1996. 25(1): p. 5-13.

15. Bouchardy, C., D.M. Parkin, and M. Khlat, Cancer mortality among Chinese and South-East Asian migrants in France. Int J Cancer, 1994. 58(5): p. 638-43.
16. Mousavi, S.M., et al., Cancer incidence among Iranian immigrants in Sweden and Iranian residents compared to the native Swedish population. European Journal of Cancer, 2010. 46(3): p. 599-605.
17. Smith, L.K., et al., Latest trends in cancer incidence among UK South Asians in Leicester. Br J Cancer, 2003. 89(1): p. 70-3.
18. Winter, H., et al., Cancer incidence in the south Asian population of England (1990-92). Br J Cancer, 1999. 79(3-4): p. 645-54.
19. Swerdlow, A.J., et al., Cancer mortality in Indian and British ethnic immigrants from the Indian subcontinent to England and Wales. Br J Cancer, 1995. 72(5): p. 1312-9.
20. Grulich, A.E., et al., Cancer mortality in African and Caribbean migrants to England and Wales. Br J Cancer, 1992. 66(5): p. 905-11.
21. Swerdlow, A., Mortality and cancer incidence in Vietnamese refugees in England and Wales: a follow-up study. Int J Epidemiol, 1991. 20(1): p. 13-9.
22. Mousavi, S.M., J. Sundquist, and K. Hemminki, Nasopharyngeal and hypopharyngeal carcinoma risk among immigrants in Sweden. Int J Cancer, 2010.
23. Stirbu, I., et al., Cancer mortality rates among first and second generation migrants in the Netherlands: Convergence toward the rates of the native Dutch population. Int J Cancer, 2006. 119(11): p. 2665-72.
24. Bouchardy, C., P. Wanner, and D.M. Parkin, Cancer mortality among sub-Saharan African migrants in France. Cancer Causes Control, 1995. 6(6): p. 539-44.
25. Winkler, V., et al., Cancer profile of migrants from the Former Soviet Union in Germany: incidence and mortality. Cancer Causes Control, 2009.
26. Hemminki, K., et al., Liver and gallbladder cancer in immigrants to Sweden. European journal of cancer (Oxford, England: 1990), 2010. 46(5): p. 926-31.
27. Arnold, M., et al., Breast and stomach cancer incidence and survival in migrants in the Netherlands, 1996-2006. Eur J Cancer Prev, 2010.
28. Hemminki, K., X.J. Li, and K. Czene, Cancer risks in first-generation immigrants to Sweden. International Journal of Cancer, 2002. 99(2): p. 218-228.
29. Andreeva, V.A., J.B. Unger, and M.A. Pentz, Breast cancer among immigrants: a systematic review and new research directions. J Immigr Minor Health, 2007. 9(4): p. 307-22.
30. Hemminki, K., et al., Preventable breast cancer is postmenopausal. Breast Cancer Res Treat, 2011. 125(1): p. 163-7.
31. Hemminki, K., X. Li, and K. Czene, Cancer risks in first-generation immigrants to Sweden. Int J Cancer, 2002. 99(2): p. 218-28.
32. Visser, O., et al., Breast cancer risk among first-generation migrants in the Netherlands. Br J Cancer, 2004. 90(11): p. 2135-7.
33. Kyobutungi, C., et al., Mortality from cancer among ethnic German immigrants from the Former Soviet Union, in Germany. Eur J Cancer, 2006. 42(15): p. 2577-84.
34. Wild, S.H., et al., Mortality from all cancers and lung, colorectal, breast and prostate cancer by country of birth in England and Wales, 2001-2003. Br J Cancer, 2006. 94(7): p. 1079-85.
35. Norredam, M., et al., Cancer incidence among 1st generation migrants compared to native Danes--a retrospective cohort study. Eur J Cancer, 2007. 43(18): p. 2717-21.

36. Mousavi, S.M., et al., Cancer incidence among Iranian immigrants in Sweden and Iranian residents compared to the native Swedish population. Eur J Cancer, 2010. 46(3): p. 599-605.

37. Harding, S. and M. Rosato, Cancer incidence among first generation Scottish, Irish, West Indian and South Asian migrants living in England and Wales. Ethn Health, 1999. 4(1-2): p. 83-92.

38. Harding, S., M. Rosato, and A. Teyhan, Trends in cancer mortality among migrants in England and Wales, 1979-2003. Eur J Cancer, 2009. 45(12): p. 2168-79.

39. Azerkan, F., et al., Risk of cervical cancer among immigrants by age at immigration and follow-up time in Sweden, from 1968 to 2004. Int J Cancer, 2008. 123(11): p. 2664-70.

40. Visser, O., et al., [Incidence of cervical cancer in women in North-Holland by country of birth from 1988-1998]. Ned Tijdschr Geneeskd, 2003. 147(2): p. 70-4.

41. Myrup, C., et al., Testicular cancer risk in first- and second-generation immigrants to Denmark. J Natl Cancer Inst, 2008. 100(1): p. 41-7.

42. Moradi, T., et al., Risk of thyroid cancer among Iranian immigrants in Sweden. Cancer Causes & Control, 2008. 19(3): p. 221-226.

43. Hemminki, K. and X.J. Li, Cancer risks in second-generation immigrants to Sweden. International Journal of Cancer, 2002. 99(2): p. 229-237.

44. Zeeb, H., et al., Transition in cancer patterns among Turks residing in Germany. Eur J Cancer, 2002. 38(5): p. 705-11.

45. Peto, J., Cancer epidemiology in the last century and the next decade. Nature, 2001. 411(6835): p. 390-5.

46. Abraido-Lanza, A.F., et al., Toward a theory-driven model of acculturation in public health research. Am J Public Health, 2006. 96(8): p. 1342-6.

3.2 Migration-sensitive cancer registration: A survey

Anna Reeske[1], Jacob Spallek[1,2]

1   University of Bremen, Bremen Institute for Prevention Research and Social Medicine,
     Germany
2   Bielefeld University, Department for Epidemiology and International Public Health,
     Germany

In the course of the MEHO-project and in order to obtain an overview of migration-sensitive data collection in the cancer setting, a survey among all European cancer registries was carried out with the support of the European Network of Cancer Registries (ENCR), Lyon [1]. A questionnaire comprising 22 questions was sent to all European cancer registries (n = 191). The questionnaire had two parts. The first part dealt with data sources, data quality (completeness, death certificate only) and the information that is collected on patient, tumour details, methods of initial treatment and outcome. The second part included questions on available data on ethnicity, nationality or migration background, data on the catchment area of the registry as well as possible or planned studies concerning immigrants.

A pre-test of the questionnaire was conducted in 11 German cancer registries of the federal states and the National Finnish Cancer Registry. In November 2007 the questionnaire was sent electronically (or as a paper version if the email address was not available) to all European cancer registries. After sending reminders the response rate was 40.8 % (fig. 3.2.1).

The data quality of the registries fits international standards based on completeness and DCO (Death Certificate Only) rate. Nearly every registry which answered reported a completeness of more than 94 % and a DCO rate of less than 5 %.

Cancer registries from all Scandinavian countries and at least one from nearly every Western Europe country answered. In addition, the majority of Eastern European countries in returned questionnaires, e.g. Belarus, Bosnia-Herzegovina, Croatia, Estonia, Latvia, Lithuania and Poland.

According to the used indicator of migrant background, the registries were classified either as "exemplary" or "less exemplary" or as "registry without any migrant-specific data." According to the MEHO definition, "exemplary" cancer registries use the individual's ethnic group (self-reported/self-assigned) or country of birth as indicator of migration background. "Less exemplary" registries use an individual's nationality or other indicators like name, religion, parents' country of birth, or the ethnic group assigned by another person, e.g. by the reporting doctor.

Several countries e.g. Italy, France and Spain maintain region-based registries instead of a nationwide registry. It turned out that no uniform method is used to assign migrant status among the respective registries.

Fig. 3.2.1: *Response in the survey conducted among European cancer registries in 2007/08*

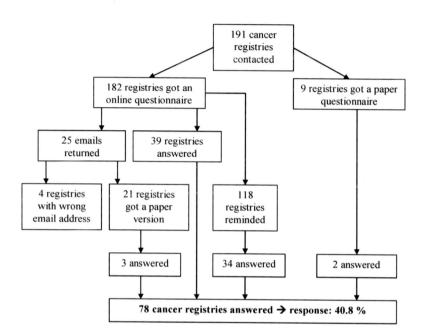

Results

Nearly half of the responding cancer registries (44.9 %) collect information on country of birth routinely (exemplary), six registries collect nationality and three collect race (less exemplary). Other information on migration background that was mentioned is the status of naturalisation.

Although a considerable proportion of surveyed cancer registries collect information on country of birth, merely 14 cancer registries reported having the possibilities to conduct migrant-specific analyses (Tab. 3.2.1). Among them, several registries explained that migrant-specific analyses would need extra resources, e.g. in terms of time and budget, but these are not available. Among the responders, merely one registry carries out routine analyses by migrant status. Additional research such as surveys or studies is carried out in 6 exemplary registries and 1 less than exemplary registry. Also, two German registries conduct additional research e.g. by record linkage procedures, because they do not obtain any migrant specific variables in their data.

Tab. 3.2.1: *Main results of the survey conducted among European cancer registries in 2007/08 (n = 78)*

	Indicator of migrant background			No migrant-specific data
	Country of birth	Nationality	Race	
Total	35 (44.9 %)	6 (7.7 %)	3 (3.8 %)	34 (43.6 %)
Possibility to conduct migrant-specific analyses				
Yes	9 (11.5 %)	0 (0.0 %)	1 (1.3 %)	4 (5.1 %)
Migrant-specific analyses actually carried out				
Routine analyses	1 (1.3 %)	0 (0.0 %)	0 (0.0 %)	0 (0.0 %)
Additional research	6 (7.7 %)	0 (0.0 %)	1 (1.3 %)	2 (2.6 %)
Numerator and denominator population available				
Yes	2 (2.6 %)	12 (15.4 %)	0 (0.0 %)	

Several registries indicated that descriptive analyses or case only/proportional analyses (e.g. Proportional Cancer Incidence Ratios, PCIRs) would be possible. For example, Turkish immigrants could be identified with the help of a name recognition software.

To summarise these results it is remarkable that nearly half of the cancer registries responded to have exemplary data, but only few conduct migrant-specific analyses. Only one register conducts such analyses routinely.

The analysis of the survey shows that currently there is a lack of data on migration status in European cancer registration and widely differing definition approaches are used. Moreover, the survey showed that even when migration status is collected, utilisation and analysis of migrant data may still be insufficient. Thus, it will be a long way to implement routine analyses. Furthermore there is still a high non-response among the European cancer registries.

After having conducted the survey, we decided to draw up "country reports" for selected countries aiming at taking a closer look at the specific potentials and problems of migrant specific analyses in European cancer registries. In detail, each country report contains a description of the specific situation with regard to (i) cancer registration, (ii) conducted studies on cancer among migrant populations, (iii) possibilities of analysing routine data or conducting dedicated studies on the cancer risks of migrants and (iv) factors, impeding the implementation of routine migrant specific analyses. These findings enable us to derive conclusions with regard to the present situation of migrant-specific cancer registration in Europe (as a whole) and its future potentials and role.

References

1. Reeske, A., J. Spallek, and O. Razum, Migrant and Ethnic Health Observatory (MEHO): Migrant-sensitive cancer registration in Europe – Results of a survey conducted among European cancer registries., in Network Eurolifestyle, Neumann G and Kirch W, Editors. 2008, Thieme Verlag: Stuttgart. p. 11-18.

Tab. 3.2.2: *Cancer Registries with the self stated possibility to conduct migrant specific analyses by exemplary and less exemplary migrant indicators*

	"Exemplary Cancer registry"	**"Less exemplary Cancer Registry"**	**"Without migrant specific variables"**
Possible to conduct migrant specific analyses	• Mallorca Cancer Registry (ES) • Modena Cancer Registry (ES) • Cancer Registry of Zaragoza (ES) • Amsterdam Cancer Registry (NL) • Netherlands Cancer Registry (NL) • Cancer Registry of the Brescia Local Health Unit (IT) • Girona Cancer Registry (IT) • Ligurian Cancer Registry (IT) • National Registry of Childhood Tumours (UK)	• Northern and Yorkshire (UK)	• Childhood Cancer Subregistry of Belarus (BY) • German Childhood Cancer Registry (DE) • Saarland Cancer Registry (DE) • Finnish Cancer Registry (FI)
Routine analyses	Swiss Childhood Cancer Registry (CH)	-	-
Additional research	• Swiss Childhood Cancer Registry (CH) • Mallorca Cancer Registry (ES) • Amsterdam Cancer Registry (NL) • Netherlands Cancer Registry (NL) • Ligurian Cancer Registry (IT) • National Registry of Childhood Tumours (UK)	• Northern and Yorkshire (UK)	• German Childhood Cancer Registry (DE) • Saarland Cancer Registry (DE)

3.3 Migration-sensitive health indicators in cancer research

Melina Arnold, Oliver Razum

Bielefeld University, Department for Epidemiology and International Public Health, Germany

Health reporting is essential in assessing and monitoring (global) health and serves as a basis for policy making. In this context, specific health indicators are helpful tools in measuring the state of (global) health, but also in recognizing trends as well as existing inequalities. In order to adequately describe the health of migrant groups, migration-sensitive health indicators need to be developed and implemented respectively.

Two major steps need to be taken in order to pave the way for migration-sensitive health and cancer research. Firstly, aiming at global comparisons, consistent definitions and identification methods in health (and cancer registration) data need to be pointed out and implemented (3.3.1). Secondly, by evaluating existing/recommended health indicators (in the cancer setting), ways to integrate migration-specific components and to conduct migration-sensitive cancer research are being suggested (3.3.2 and 3.3.3), also drawing attention to specific biases that may occur in migrant studies (3.3.4). Lastly, an overall bottom line of the both challenging and promising implementation of migration-sensitive health indicators is being delineated.

3.3.1 The challenge of identifying migrants in health and cancer registry data

Ethnicity is a social construct, referring to one's sense of identity in a cultural group or society that is sometimes hard to grasp. Unlike race, ethnicity is not restricted to phenotypes and is motivated by sharing certain views, lifestyles and cultural habits. Migrants often represent ethnic minority groups in their countries of residence and share cultural identities as well as common ideals and goals. Due to their various origins, migrant groups are often characterized by a high degree of heterogeneity which makes their adequate identification and consideration in research even more challenging. Not only the lack of consistent definitions of the migrant status, but also often missing information in most routine data sources emphasize the necessity of changing practice. Migration and cultural diversity is gaining social importance and therefore makes monitoring culturally diverse health care needs indispensible in order to ensure the supply of high quality and appropriate health care.[1]

Different concepts of ethnicity, race and migration inevitably lead to different research angles and also have an impact on how to acquire and analyse data respectively. Whereas race is mostly used to investigate the association between genetic differences and outcomes, the concept of a migration background is often applied in the course of etiologic research questions. Ethnicity on the other hand is more related to disease perception and health behaviours. Nevertheless, most countries have their own tradition of collecting the one or the other and researchers are often forced to work with what they get.

Yet, the most accepted ways of identifying and describing a migration background are to collect data on (self-assigned) ethnicity or country of birth, which also has its pitfalls but is – according to the MEHO project (see chapter 3.2) – considered exemplary. Alternatively, other ethnicity proxies such as nationality, name, religion, parental country of birth or ethnicity assigned by another person (e.g. by the doctor) can be applied to take culturally related aspects into account. The latter approaches are – again, based on our survey – considered less than exemplary and are often used when other information on ethnicity is missing.

Ethnicity (self-assigned)

Using self-assigned ethnicity as the defining indicator represents the most valid way of investigating the impact of ethnicity on health. Its concept emphasises the common sense of identity and allows conclusions regarding cultural and lifestyle-related factors.

However, this approach is also coupled with limitations that mainly refer to the test-retest reliability. Self-perceived ethnicity may vary over time and may be dependent on the level of integration in the host country. In addition, the assessment of this variable may be extremely challenging: whether to use predefined categories or an open question is dependent on the study question and the degree of heterogeneity that is aimed at. Furthermore, the exact wording of a question on ethnic identification is essential for the reliability of the answers. It is also important to take multiple generations of migrants into consideration. A migrant background may go far back in time and generation assignment may not always be possible. Defining migrants on the basis of their self-perceived ethnicity is exemplary and an already adopted method in some countries (e.g. the United Kingdom), although it can sometimes be difficult to grasp and may range from biological concepts through the national origin (of the persons or ancestors to cultural affiliation. It can thus make international comparisons challenging [1-3].

Country of birth (own or parental)

The usage of country of birth as a proxy for ethnicity is widespread and emphasises the aspect of descent or common geographical origin. It is often routinely collected for administrative purposes and therefore likely to be available in many registries. It is an objective and unchanging attribute, but remains a crude measure that does not allow for distinctions with regard to ethnic diversity within migrant groups. Many countries host more than one ethnicity: Surinamese Creoles (with descendants from West Africa) and Hindoestanen (with descendants from South Asia), two very different groups, mostly born in Suriname and of Dutch nationality, can for instance not be distinguished using the country of birth approach. The lack of heterogeneity and validity (no gold standard available) plays an important role in this case. An advantage of this approach is that migrants can clearly be distinguished from their direct offspring (sometimes called "second generation") if the individual and parental country of birth is available. However, this method becomes inaccurate over the generations, and already the "third generation" cannot be identified using this method (as long as the country of birth of the grandparents is not available). Yet its application in research settings is simple and can be done by an outsider. It is therefore considered to be more objective and constant than self-perceived ethnicity [2, 4].

Nationality

Nationality as a proxy for migrant status is probably the most simple, objectively assessable and convenient method because it is universally available and applicable. It is though a very crude measure, and in many countries it is not reliable anymore. Nationality is a characteristic that may change over time (uptake of citizenship of host country, marriage, etc), and it has only a weak link to the ethnic background. Since the legislation to obtain a new nationality is different between countries, the comparability of data can be problematic. Moreover, many people originating from former European colonies hold European citizenships, but have different ethnic origins. Also, the rate of naturalization among former labour migrants is increasing. All these issues make nationality a crude proxy for ethnicity, although it is in many countries the only available identifier.

Name

Name-based approaches are can be applied needing no other information but names and have for instance been used for Turks in Germany [5-6] and South Asians in the United Kingdom [7]. It is only feasible with a limited number of migrant groups and does not provide any information regarding actual migration, generation and ethnic identity. Using this method, identification of migrants is carried out based on a set of family and first names that need to be distinct and unique for the country of origin. For example, Turkish names (in Turkey) usually have a meaning in the Turkish language and are free of religious content. They can therefore easily be distinguished from Arabic names [6]. After a automatic part of the applied algorithm, experts need to be involved in the analysis in order to verify the results. However, this method slowly loses its validity due to intercultural marriages, increasing naturalization and rapidly growing ethnic diversity that cannot be appreciated by using the name as an ethnicity proxy. Data privacy regulations may also inhibit this method since very sensitive information in clear text is needed to for the conduct.

Other (additional) indicators

Other common proxies for ethnicity are religion, language spoken, migration history and ethnicity assigned by another person. However, these most often serve as additional discrimination factors in order to compensate for the limitations of other identifiers or to improve their validity respectively. Spoken language can for example be used in order to amend the country of birth identifier and thus to improve the way of appropriately capturing a complex migration background.

Which approach to chose is mostly based on the availability of data and the actual research question respectively. For this reason, it is highly context- and country-dependent when it comes to the use of an identifier variable for migration and its validity. Prospectively, in order to achieve comparability and to allow for cross-country analyses, it is important to implement comprehensive, exemplary and unique identifiers, such as a standardized definition of ethnicity or consistent usage of country of birth.

3.3.2 Health quality indicators in cancer research

In order to increase and ensure accessibility and quality of cancer care, irrespective of socioeconomic position or ethnic background, effective health information and monitoring are essential. Several organisations acting on the European and international level are dedicated to systematic data gathering, analysis, interpretation and dissemination, eventually being shared for evidence-based health policies and in order to develop comparative health information.

Standardized health indicators are vital for national as well as international comparisons and may explain cross-country variations in outcomes. Health indicators are based on (future) needs and aims and are mostly defined on what is available in the specific country. After drafting a long-term framework and developing country-specific implementation plans, evidence-based measures can be launched.

ECHIM (European Community Health Indicators and Monitoring), a project initiated by the European Commission, built on the work of ECHI (European Community Health Indicators), aims at helping countries to implement, collect and disseminate health indicators, based on the ECHI shortlist of 88 indicators. In cancer research, important indicators that reflect quality of care have been developed in the course of various projects. Most prominent, apart from those of ECHIM, are the Health Care Quality Indicators (HCQI) by the Organisation for Economic Co-operation and Development (OECD) and the European Cancer Health Indicator Project (EUROCHIP). Table 3.3.1 provides an overview of all

Tab. 3.3.1: Health quality indicators in cancer research

Indicator	Suggested by	Description
Cancer mortality (rates, trends, projections, PYLL*)	**ECHIM, HCQI, EUROCHIP**	All-cancer mortality and mortality of the most important cancers (breast, cervical, colon, lung and prostate cancer), per 100.000 population, in a given year (crude and age-standardized). Calculated as the number of patients that died of cancer during the given calendar year divided by person-years at risk (stratified by sex, geographical area, period and age group).
Cancer incidence (rates, trends and projections)	**ECHIM item 20, EUROCHIP**	Corresponds to the all-cancer incidence and incidence of the most important cancers (per 100.000 persons) in a given year. The numerator is the number of patients with newly diagnosed cancer during the given calendar year, divided by the denominator (background population), person-years at risk (per sex, geographical area, period and age group), expressed as per 100.000 population.
Breast, cervical, colorectal cancer screening	**ECHIM items 58-60, HCQI**	Proportion of persons in the screening age group (breast cancer: 50-69; cervical cancer: 20-69; colorectal cancer: 50-74) reporting to have undergone a cancer screening test within the past two (breast and colorectal cancer) or three (cervical cancer) years.
Cancer (relative) survival rates (breast, cervix, colorectal)	**ECHIM item 78, HCQI, EUROCHIP**	Relative cancer survival corresponds to the proportion of patients who survive at least five years after diagnosis, after correction for background mortality.
Cancer treatment quality	**ECHIM item 83, EUROCHIP**	Compliance with best oncology practice
Stage at cancer diagnosis	**EUROCHIP**	Extension of tumour at diagnosis, usually indicated with clinical and pathological TNM status. Percentage of cases with early diagnosis and cases with a metastatic test.
Cancer palliative therapy	**EUROCHIP**	Use of morphine in cancer patients, percentage of patients receiving palliative radiotherapy
Cancer treatment delay	**EUROCHIP**	The average time (in days) between the date of first treatment and the pre-diagnostic date, by cancer site (breast, colon and rectal cancer).
Coverage/ completeness of cancer registration	**EUROCHIP**	Population covered by high quality cancer registries

*Person-years-of-life-lost

Tab. 3.3.1 (continued)

Data source(s)	Migration–related research questions
Population-based cancer and cause of death registries; secondary data sources (GLOBOCAN)	Do cancer mortality patterns differ between migrants and non-migrants? Are there changes over time/across migrant generations?
Population-based cancer registries; secondary data sources (GLOBO-CAN)	Is there a difference in underlying risk factor patterns that causes disparities in cancer incidence? Are there changes over time/across migrant generations?
EUROSTAT and OECD (available every five years)	Does uptake/attendance of preventive measures differ between migrant and indigenous populations? What are the main problems/barriers?
EUROCARE, cancer registries (delay of 2-5 yrs)	Does survival differ between migrants and non-migrants? Which factors play a role?
Hospitals	Are migrants treated differently and does that have an impact on their survival/mortality?
Population-based cancer registries	Is there a difference at stage at diagnosis, resulting in differences in mortality/survival?
Hospitals	Do therapy measures differ?
Cancer registries – still to be developed due to some modifications that might be necessary.	Is there a difference in the time span between actions/treatments between migrants and non-migrants (possibly resulting in differences in mortality/survival?)?
IARC	How complete is the registration of variables needed to identify migrant populations?

health quality indicators in cancer research recommended and developed during the course of the above mentioned projects. Furthermore, migration-related research questions underline the relevance of each indicator. Promoting the comprehensive collection of these indicators is the basis for developing ways to involve migration-sensitive components (see Tab. 3.3.2, p. 50).

3.3.3 Conducting migration-sensitive cancer research

Most cancer registries do not routinely collect data on ethnicity or they have insufficient completeness of this variable. This has also been confirmed by the MEHO survey (see chapter 3.2). But even if migrant-sensitive data is not directly available in the registries, other methods can be applied to conduct migrant-sensitive research such as linkage procedures given that (a proxy of) ethnicity is included in other databases (like population data from statistical offices or medical records) or by using name based approaches. In order to be able to analyse health quality indicators in a migration-sensitive setting, the following steps help exploring ways for their implementation. How to construct the numerator (identifying migrants)

The numerator comprises (incident) cancer cases according to sex, age, geographical area and period. Of course, migrants need to be identified using a variable indicating ethnicity or a proxy respectively. Ways to identify migrants in cancer registry data and their validity have been discussed previously (see 3.3.1).

How to construct the denominator (choosing the reference population)

The denominator, defining the background population under risk, has to cover the same catchment area as the numerator (population or regional level) and needs to take into account the same time period. Furthermore, exactly the same definition of ethnicity needs to be applied as well as matching data quality, completeness, sensitivity and specificity of the used method. Data on the background population can in most cases be obtained from statistical offices or population registries. A common problem is that the definitions of migrant status in the numerator and in the denominator do not match.

How to merge numerator and denominator and perform migrant-specific analyses

Different methods can be applied in order to merge numerator and denominator, strongly depending on the availability, conceivableness and type of data obtained.

Direct methods

The most straight-forward way to perform migrant-specific analyses is to identify migrants directly in the data of the cancer registry (nominator) and to acquire data on the background population (denominator) based on the same definitions and categories. This simple record linkage is possible for instance on the basis of names, date of birth or even more convenient using a personal identifier or health service number that has already been introduced in some countries.

Indirect methods: linkage

Technically more complex options are linkage procedures that can be applied if no information on ethnicity is available in cancer registry data. Given that ethnicity is included in other databases such as population census data, data from general register offices or (cause of) death databases, these records can be linked to health data (like hospital discharge or cancer registry data) using probability matching procedures. An advantage is the availability of a personalised identifier like the Community Health Index (CHI) in Scotland [8] or the Citizen Service Number (CSN) that has been introduced in the Netherlands and is obligatory as well as unique for every person making use of the national health care system. Using this approach, anonymised data merging can be achieved by applying data encryption methods. In a recent study, Bhopal and colleagues [9] successfully demonstrated that linking databases can provide solid migration-sensitive cancer data without recourse to cohort studies. Furthermore, this method is in principal internationally applicable, although data privacy regulations may vary and always deserve strict adherence.

Indirect methods: name-based approaches

An additional indirect method to conduct migrant-sensitive analyses are name-based approaches where the same procedure of identifying migrants is applied to both the numerator (cancer registry data) and the denominator population (reference population). This has for instance been performed in Germany [10], the Netherlands [11] and the United Kingdom [12-13].

Numerator-only migrant-specific analyses

Alternatively, given that linkage is not feasible or possible, numerator-only based analyses/measures can be used to perform migrant-specific analyses. Options are for example Proportional Cancer Incidence Ratios (PCIR) [14-16] or calculating relative survival using the corresponding background mortality (life tables) [17].

3.3.4 Bias in migrant studies (the cancer setting)

Identification methods

The method of identifying migrants can lead to substantial bias with regard to ethnic identity and variations within migrant groups (see also 3.3.1). Country of birth, the currently most accepted proxy for ethnicity [4], does not address these issues and can therefore lead to considerable misclassifications as well as under-estimations of mortality differences. Ideally, risk variations within migrant groups can be taken into account by stratification for additional culturally-related factors such as mother tongue and exact birth place. In some cases, adjustments for socioeconomic position may also help distinguishing certain groups. [18-19]

In this context, one should also give special attention to matching numerator and denominator figures when identifying migrant groups. It is essential that migrant status is defined in an identical manner in both cases and reference population

Selection effects

Migrants are often likely to be a non-random, self-selected group of the population of their country of origin [20]. This can for instance be reflected in particular (limited) geographical areas of origin or certain cultural or social groups with own distinctive cancer patterns [2]. Seeking a new life requires energy and resources, leading to selective migration of particularly healthy individuals and resulting in favorable health outcomes in the new host country. This health selection effect (*healthy migrant effect*), accountable for an initial advantage in health, only affects first generation migrants from specific countries (primarily low-income countries) and has been reported to decrease over time [21]. Work-related selection (*healthy worker effect*) might be another explanation for lower incidence and mortality figures [22].

In studies, this bias can be explored by investigating cancer risk according to duration of stay in the host country and taking into account age at migration. Significant changes in cancer risk between the population of the host country and recent migrant groups may be precipitated by this form of bias. Yet, it can be questionable how strong the healthy migrant effect is, because most migrants migrate at an age at which symptoms of the major causes of death/ chronic conditions are rarely present. [2]

A second important selection effect concerns the selective remigration of a diseased or unhealthy subgroup of migrants, leaving a healthier selection of their population in the host country. This so called *salmon bias* assumes that migrant groups are more likely to return to their country of origin when they become elderly or chronically ill and therefore quantifies the impact of deaths abroad. This often unregistered remigration leads to inaccurate denominator figures, resulting in a seemingly better survival and lower mortality of migrants in the host country [22-24].

However, there is evidence for remaining health and mortality advantages after accounting for the above mentioned selection effects, remaining a paradox but pointing to the concept of health transition [25]. As migrants from less developed regions migrate to more affluent countries, they retain the disease risk patterns typical for their country of origin, where infectious diseases often still dominate and chronic conditions such as cancer are only slowly in the ascendant. It may therefore take many years till mortality patterns diverge towards those of the population of the host country respectively. [26]

Social and behavioral factors (confounding)

In the United States, ethnicity is often used as a socioeconomic indicator, whereas in other countries, socioeconomic circumstances are used to approximate ethnicity. The problems of these approaches are obvious and the need to analyze ethnicity and socioeconomic position as separate variables in health studies has been recognized [27].

Socioeconomic position is a strong determinant for cancer risk and can also potentially explain some aspects of ethnic variation in cancer risk. A certain degree of interaction between low socioeconomic status (SES) and ethnicity has been proven (migrants tend to be socially disadvantaged in the host country), but what exactly the separate effect of ethnicity on cancer risk is, often remains unclear. SES is often taken into account using ecological measures which are sometimes limited with regard to their validity for all ethnic groups. Some studies found that the size of socioeconomic inequalities varies between ethnic groups, but that socioeconomic differences are larger in the population of the host country [19, 27]. SES should thus – if possible – be included as an important covariable in any analysis. In any case, one should be aware and carefully distinguish ethnic and socioeconomic inequalities and find a way to disentangle the two concepts.

Differences in cancer risk may also partly be attributable to ethnic variation with respect to social support and social gradients in behavioral risk factor patterns. Social support can in some ethnic groups be a key factor, determining socioeconomic disparities within ethnic groups. High levels of support, e.g. close family ties and strong group cohesions, may partly avert adverse effects of a low socioeconomic background.

Lifestyle and behavioral risk factors may persist or change over time. Migration especially entails completely new, compelling exposures, often leading to an adoption of unhealthy Western lifestyles in migrant groups. The currently high prevalence of smokers among mainly male migrants residing in more affluent countries for instance reflects their tendency to adopt behavior common in the host country. [28]

Migrants tend to settle in certain (often urban) areas. It thus needs to be considered carefully which comparisons between migrants and the population of the host country are appropriate and most reasonable.

Many cancer registries already routinely collect a broad range of demographic variables that can also be considered important determinants (confounders) in migration-sensitive cancer research (e.g. date of diagnosis/death, marital status, place of residence, ethnic group/ country of birth, occupation, SES). Nevertheless, data on behavioral patterns is often missing or incomplete.

Data quality

There is often considerable disparity between countries in the accuracy of the coded underlying cause of death (differences in access to diagnosis facilities, manners of completing and coding death certificates, etc.) and often also in the quality, completeness and coverage of cancer registry data.

When including data from the migrants' country of origin and conducting comparisons with the host country, differences in the ascertainment of some cancers, especially those with diagnostic difficulties, can be even more grave. It can lead to a so called "*overshoot*", a phenomenon giving rise to higher rates in migrants compared with the host country, but lower rates compared with the country of origin. Furthermore, rates in the host country can be influenced by the detection of asymptomatic cancers during screening, surgery or autopsy. [2]

The quality of cancer registry data can be assessed by comparing certain indices e.g. proportions of deaths certified with non-specific causes, cancer deaths at ill-defined sites and other traditional quality indicators (e.g. percentage histologically verified, death-certificate-only cases or the ratio of mortality to incidence) [29].

Suggested web-based resources

Indicators

• **ECHIM** (European Community Health Indicators Monitoring): (http:// www. echim.org/)
• **EUROCHIP** (European Cancer Health Indicator Project): (http://www. tumori.net/eurochip/)
• Eurostat

- **OECD** (Organisation for Economic Co-operation and Development): Health Care Quality Indicators (**HCQI**) (http://www.oecd.org/health/hcqi).

Cancer Data

- **GLOBOCAN 2008** (global cancer incidence and mortality data): (http://globocan.iarc.fr/)
- **EUROCARE** (European Cancer-Registry-based study on survival and care of cancer patients): (http://www.eurocare.it/)

Institutions/Organizations

- **ENCR** (European Network of Cancer Registries): (http://www.encr.com.fr/)
- EUROCADET:(http://www.eurocadet.org/index.php)
- **EUROSTAT** (Statistics on the EU and candidate countries): (http://epp.eurostat.ec.europa.eu/portal/page/portal/eurostat/home/)
- **IARC** (International Agency for Research on Cancer): (http://www.iarc.fr/)
- **IACR** (International Associations of Cancer Registries): (http://www.iacr.com.fr/)
- **WHO** (World Health Organization), Cancer: (http://www.who.int/cancer/en/)

References

1. Bhopal, R.S., Ethnicity, Race, and Health in Multicultural Societies: Foundations for Better Epidemiology, Public Health, and Health Care. 2007: Oxford Univ Pr.
2. Parkin, D.M. and M. Khlat, Studies of cancer in migrants: rationale and methodology. Eur J Cancer, 1996. 32A(5): p. 761-71.
3. Bhopal, R., Glossary of terms relating to ethnicity and race: for reflection and debate. J Epidemiol Community Health, 2004. 58(6): p. 441-5.
4. Stronks, K., I. Kulu-Glasgow, and C. Agyemang, The utility of 'country of birth' for the classification of ethnic groups in health research: the Dutch experience. Ethn Health, 2009. 14(3): p. 1-14.
5. Razum, O., et al., Combining a name algorithm with a capture-recapture method to retrieve cases of Turkish descent from a German population-based cancer registry. European journal of cancer (Oxford, England: 1990), 2000. 36(18): p. 2380-4.
6. Razum, O., H. Zeeb, and S. Akgun, How useful is a name-based algorithm in health research among Turkish migrants in Germany? Tropical medicine & international health: TM & IH, 2001. 6(8): p. 654-61.
7. Nitsch, D., et al., Validation and utility of a computerized South Asian names and group recognition algorithm in ascertaining South Asian ethnicity in the national renal registry. QJM: monthly journal of the Association of Physicians, 2009. 102(12): p. 865-72.
8. Fischbacher, C.M., et al., Record linked retrospective cohort study of 4.6 million people exploring ethnic variations in disease: myocardial infarction in South Asians. BMC Public Health, 2007. 7: p. 142.
9. Bhopal, R., et al., Cohort profile: Scottish Health and Ethnicity Linkage Study of 4.65 million people exploring ethnic variations in disease in Scotland. Int J Epidemiol, 2010.

10. Spallek, J., et al., Cancer incidence rate ratios of Turkish immigrants in Hamburg, Germany: A registry based study. Cancer epidemiology, 2009. 33(6): p. 413-8.
11. Bouwhuis, C.B. and H.A. Moll, Determination of ethnicity in children in The Netherlands: two methods compared. Eur J Epidemiol, 2003. 18(5): p. 385-8.
12. Nanchahal, K., et al., Development and validation of a computerized South Asian Names and Group Recognition Algorithm (SANGRA) for use in British health-related studies. Journal of public health medicine, 2001. 23(4): p. 278-85.
13. dos Santos Silva, I., et al., Survival from breast cancer among South Asian and non-South Asian women resident in South East England. Br J Cancer, 2003. 89(3): p. 508-12.
14. Zeeb, H., et al., Transition in cancer patterns among Turks residing in Germany. Eur J Cancer, 2002. 38(5): p. 705-11.
15. Spallek, J., et al., Cancer patterns among children of Turkish descent in Germany: a study at the German Childhood Cancer Registry. BMC Public Health, 2008. 8: p. 152.
16. Breslow, N.E. and N.E. Day, Statistical methods in cancer research. Volume II--The design and analysis of cohort studies. IARC Sci Publ, 1987(82): p. 1-406.
17. Spix, C., et al., Cancer survival among children of Turkish descent in Germany 1980-2005: a registry-based analysis. BMC Cancer, 2008. 8: p. 355.
18. McCormack, V.A., et al., Heterogeneity of breast cancer risk within the South Asian female population in England: a population-based case-control study of first-generation migrants. Br J Cancer, 2004. 90(1): p. 160-6.
19. Bos, V., et al., Socioeconomic inequalities in mortality within ethnic groups in the Netherlands, 1995-2000. J Epidemiol Community Health, 2005. 59(4): p. 329-35.
20. Marmot, M., Changing places changing risks: the study of migrants. Public Health Rev, 1993. 21(3-4): p. 185-95.
21. Stirbu, I., et al., Cancer mortality rates among first and second generation migrants in the Netherlands: Convergence toward the rates of the native Dutch population. Int J Cancer, 2006. 119(11): p. 2665-72.
22. Razum, O., et al., Low overall mortality of Turkish residents in Germany persists and extends into a second generation: merely a healthy migrant effect? Tropical medicine & international health: TM & IH, 1998. 3(4): p. 297-303.
23. Bos, V., et al., Ethnic inequalities in age- and cause-specific mortality in The Netherlands. Int J Epidemiol, 2004. 33(5): p. 1112-9.
24. Marmot, M.G., A.M. Adelstein, and L. Bulusu, Lessons from the study of immigrant mortality. Lancet, 1984. 1(8392): p. 1455-7.
25. Razum, O., H. Zeeb, and S. Rohrmann, The 'healthy migrant effect'--not merely a fallacy of inaccurate denominator figures. Int J Epidemiol, 2000. 29(1): p. 191-2.
26. Razum, O. and D. Twardella, Time travel with Oliver Twist--towards an explanation foa a paradoxically low mortality among recent immigrants. Trop Med Int Health, 2002. 7(1): p. 4-10.
27. Smith, G.D., Learning to live with complexity: ethnicity, socioeconomic position, and health in Britain and the United States. Am J Public Health, 2000. 90(11): p. 1694-8.
28. Reeske, A., J. Spallek, and O. Razum, Changes in smoking prevalence among first- and second-generation Turkish migrants in Germany – an analysis of the 2005 Microcensus. Int J Equity Health, 2009. 8: p. 26.
29. Schmidtmann, I. and M. Blettner, How Do Cancer Registries in Europe Estimate Completeness of Registration? Methods Inf Med, 2009. 3: p. 267-271.

Chapter 4:

Country Reports

4. Country Reports

4.1 Finland

Eero Pukkala[1], Anna Reeske[2]

1   Finnish Cancer Registry, Institute for Statistical and Epidemiological Cancer Research
    Helsinki, Finland
2   University of Bremen, Bremen Institute for Prevention Research and Social Medicine,
    Germany

4.1.1 General information about Finland

Finland has a total area of 338,424 km², but along with Norway and Iceland it is the most sparsely populated country in Europe. The population amounts to about 5.4 million at the end of 2009 [1], corresponding to an average population density of 15 inhabitants per square kilometre [2]. The majority of Finnish inhabitants are living in urban areas, mostly in the Southwest of Finland (about 64%). About one million is living in the capital area of Helsinki.

The majority of Finns speak Finnish, but there is a Swedish speaking minority in Finland of about 5%. Finland belonged to the Swedish Kingdom from the 13th to the early 19th century. The Sami people, also are referred to as Lapps, represent one of the indigenous populations in Finland. Nowadays the number of Sami is assumed to be about 7,500, mostly living in the very north of Finland. This group is characterized by a specific genetic background and has had a way of life that differs from the other Finns [3].

Population

At the end of 2009, Finland had a population size of 5,351,000, with 49.1% men and 50.9% women [1]. There has been an increase of immigration during the past twenty years, leading to a positive net migration. Most of the migrants in Finland are from neighbouring countries such as the Russian Federation and Estonia (work-migration), but in the last decades there has also been increased migration of war refugees. In 1988 a comparatively small number of 9,700 persons from foreign countries immigrated to Finland, in 2000 the number was 16,800 and thus increased by 74.1%. Up to 2008, the number of immigrants from other EU countries coming to Finland grew continuously since 1997 (Fig. 4.1.1) and in the past eight years this number even exceeded the number of emigrated persons from Finland to other EU countries. In addition, the number of migrants from abroad contributed more to the increase of Finland's population in 2008 than its natural growth [1].

In 2009, Finland's number of new immigrants decreased for the first time since 2000. In this year, Finland registered 26,700 new arrivals, a decrease of 2,400 persons compared to the immigration number in 2008 [4].

Fig. 4.1.1: *Migration between Finland and other countries 1988-2009, based on data from [5]*

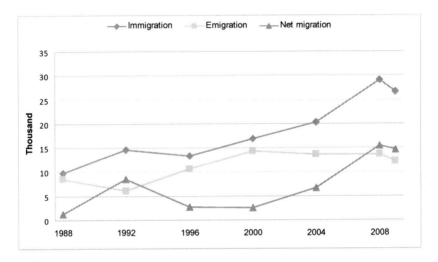

Population according to country of birth and citizenship

Finland has a very small proportion of foreign citizens (2.9%=155,705 persons), the seventh lowest among all EU 27 countries [1]. Within this group of foreign citizens 139,647 (89.7%) were born abroad and 16,058 (10.3%) were born in Finland. In both groups the majority speaks a native language different from the three official ones (Finnish, Swedish, Sami).

Among persons with a Finnish citizenship, the vast majority was both born in Finland and speaks Finnish as native language. Among the persons born abroad with a Finnish citizenship, the majority are foreign-language speakers (Fig. 4.1.2).

In 2009, the majority of foreign citizens were Russian (18.1%) and Estonian (16.4%) (Tab. 4.1.1). Further groups held citizenships from Sweden, Somalia, China, Thailand, Germany, Turkey, Iraq and UK [4].

Population according to native language

The majority of Finland's population speaks Finnish (90.7%) and Swedish (5.4%) as their native language. Furthermore, people speaking any of the three Sami languages (0.03%) have the right to use their language in official situa-

Fig. 4.1.2: *Population of Finland according to country of birth, citizenship and native language 31.12.2009, adapted from [1]*

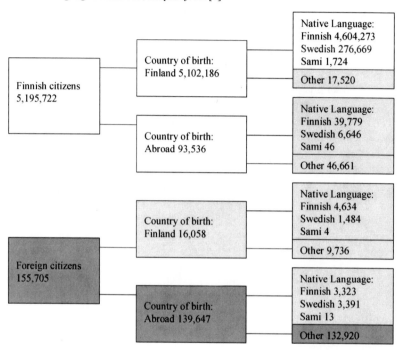

Tab. 4.1.1 *Foreigners in Finland according to country of citizenship [1]*

Country of citizenship	2008	%	Annual change (%)	2009	%	Annual change (%)
Russian Federation	26,909	18.8	2.7	28,210	18.1	4.8
Estonia	22,604	15.8	13.0	25,510	16.4	12.9
Sweden	8,439	5.9	1.1	8,506	5.5	0.8
Somalia	4,919	3.4	1.4	5,570	3.6	13.2
China	4,620	3.2	16.1	5,180	3.3	12.1
Thailand	3,932	2.7	13.3	4,497	2.9	14.4
Iraq	3,238	2.3	6.7	3,978	2.6	22.9
Turkey	3,429	2.4	7.8	3,809	2.4	11.1
Germany	3,502	2.4	5.5	3,628	2.3	3.6
United Kingdom	3,213	2.2	2.2	3,333	2.1	3.7
Others	58,451	40.8	9.9	63,484	40.8	8.6
Total	**143,256**	**100**	**7.9**	**155,705**	**100**	**8.7**

tions. The number of persons with a native language other than Finnish, Swedish or Sami has doubled over the past 9 years and exceeded 200,000 in 2009 (3.9%). In 2009, the largest groups by foreign native language were Russian, Estonian, English, Somali and Arabic.

Population registration in Finland: The Population Information System

Statistics Finland is responsible for compiling statistics on the conditions of the society, including demographics. Since 1975, statistics on the population structure are mainly derived from the *Population Information System* maintained by the Population Register Centre in cooperation with the local register offices. The Population Register Centre was founded in 1969 and operates under the Ministry of Finance. The Population Information System comprises a computerised national register that contains basic data on Finnish and foreign citizens permanently residing in Finland. It is based on the latest population registration that has been carried out in 1989 and the changes that have been notified continuously since then [6].

The Population Information System contains information on:

- Name
- Personal identity code (including information on date of birth and sex)
- Address
- Citizenship
- Native language
- Family relations
- Date of death, date and country of immigration/emigration
- Residential history
- Buildings (building code, location, owner, area, facilities and network connections, intended use and year of construction)
- Real estate (real estate unit identifier, owner's name and address, and buildings located on the property).

Personal identity code

For registration purposes, all Finnish citizens (born in Finland or abroad) are allocated a personal identity code (PID) that remains unchanged throughout lifetime. The PID consists of eleven digits: The first six digits indicate the day, month and year of birth followed by a symbol indicating the century of birth, an individual three-digit running number among those born on the same day (odd number for men and even number for women) and a control character (number or letter, out of a selection of 31 characters).

People born in Finland are automatically assigned a PID from the Population Information Register based on the birth certification.

Persons with a foreign citizenship who migrated to Finland and intend to obtain a permanent residence (in addition to those who stayed for more than one year) are also assigned a PID. It is not possible to live in Finland without PID as it is necessary for the payment of wages, salaries, fees, and pensions, in bank transactions, to open a bank account, to visit hospital etc. [6].

Availability of information on migration background

In terms of relevant variables for describing a migration background, the Finnish Population Register contains information on citizenship, country of birth and native language of each registered person. The three determinants are described in the following paragraphs extracted from a description published by Statistics Finland [1]:

> "**Citizenship** refers to a legislative bond between an individual and the State defining the individual's status in the State as well as the basic rights and duties existing between the individual and the State (Nationality Act, 359/2003). Persons with both Finnish and foreign citizenship will be entered in the statistics as Finnish nationals. If a foreign national living in Finland has several nationalities, that person will be entered in the statistics as a national of the country on whose passport he or she arrived in the country."

> "Country of birth is determined on the basis of the mother's permanent home country at the time of birth. This means, for example, that the country of birth of Estonian immigrants born before Estonian independence is the Soviet Union. Similarly, the country of birth of people who were born in areas that Finland has subsequently ceded is Finland even though the area no longer is Finnish territory. The country of birth is indicated according to the form of government at the time of birth."

> "**Language** is recorded in the Population Information System at the same time as parents register the name and religious denomination of their newborn. That language will be changed only upon separate application. For those babies born at the end of the year, for whom no name, language and religion have been registered in the Population Information System during January, the mother's language and religion are entered in the statistics for the end of the year. For the next year's statistics this information has become revised once notifications have been received. Language for children of bi- or multilingual families can be changed in the Population Information System."

All three concepts are used to create statistics on Finland's population structure by Statistics Finland.

4.1.2 The Finnish Health Care System

Finland consists of 342 municipalities (2010) that vary to a high degree in terms of population number and structure (e.g. number of inhabitants, age structure) as well as regarding the use of health care services and expenditure. Hence, Finland has a largely decentralized health care system. Decisions on structure and planning of the health care system are made on the municipal level and are realised by a health committee, the municipal council and the municipal executive board (Fig. 5). Each municipality belongs to one central hospital district, which form the five university hospital districts in Finland.

The majority of total health care costs are financed by municipalities mainly through the municipal fixed income tax. Further, about 18% are financed by the state, 15% by the National Health Insurance (NHI) and about 24% by private sources [7]. The NHI is statutory for all permanent residents in Finland. It is run by the Social Insurance Institution and mainly covers the use of private services.

Primary health care services are available for all residents in Finland, irrespective of financial situation, citizenship or place of residence. Primary health care as well as prevention services are usually provided by municipal health centres. Offered services include, for example, maternity and child care, prevention, dental care, and general outpatient care. Some centres also include an inpatient department for patients with chronic diseases [8].

Private health care only accounts for a small proportion of the total health care expenditure and includes occupational health care services. The municipal health care system and the private health care system are not mutually exclusive. For example municipal centres may contract private practitioners for special services [8].

4.1.3 Cancer registration in Finland

First cancer incidence statistics in Finland were collected in 1910, and in 1939-1940 there was another short period of cancer data collection, however discontinued because of the World War Two. The current registration system was initiated in 1952. Finland has one central cancer register, Finnish Cancer Registry (FCR), that covers the whole country and that is responsible for all aspects of registration. The FCR holds the database currently containing more than one million cancer cases diagnosed in Finland since 1953. In 2008, more than 27,000 new invasive cancer cases were reported to the FCR, 13,700 in males (incidence rate, adjusted for age to the Word standard population: 286/100,000) and 13,700 new cases in females (IR: 250/100,000) [9]. In addition, thousands of basal cell carcinomas, borderline malignancies and precancerous lesions are registered every year.

Registration procedure in the FCR

All health care facilities (physicians, hospitals and pathological laboratories) that diagnose a treat a new cancer case are obligated to report it to the FCR by using a standard notification form or data records with similar contents. Nowadays, the majority of notifications are sent electronically. Also, Statistics Finland annually reports all cancer cases mentioned in the death certificates by sending a computerised file. All dates and causes of death (also non-cancer deaths) of deceased cancer patients are inserted in the FCR database by linking the two databases through the patient's individual PID. The PID is used for case identification in nearly all processes of registration. It also allows a precise follow-up of cancer patients.

The following diseases have to be reported to the Registry:
- All malignant neoplasms (e.g. carcinomas (also basaliomas), sarcomas, malignant lymphomas, leukaemias, multiple myeloma, gliomas, melanoma, etc.);
- Carcinoid tumours, pheochromocytomas, thymomas, ameloblastomas, and chordomas; Carcinoma in situ lesions (except those of the skin);
- CIN III and CIL III of the cervix uteri; histologically benign tumours of the central nervous system and meninges, transitional cell papillomas of the urinary tract, and ovarian tumours with borderline malignancy.

Each primary tumour that is diagnosed as an independent one is registered separately and coded as a separate entity in the FCR database.

During the process of data entry and coding, quality checks are carried out to identify non-existent codes and code combinations as well as implausible data. In the case of implausible or missing data, physicians and hospitals are requested to check or add the information. For quality check purposes, the FCR database is also regularly linked with the Central Population Register, e.g. to check the PIDs or to add information on official name, place of residence, and possible dates of emigration and death.

Final coding of cancer data is done by qualified secretaries and supervised by the FCR chief physician. For diagnostic coding of the primary cancer site a modified version of ICD-7 was used for cases diagnosed before 2006, but have been later translated to codes of the third edition of ICD-O. For cases diagnosed in 2007 or later, original coding is done according to ICD-O-3.

Completeness and accuracy of data

The completeness and accuracy of the FCR data are among the best in the world. More than 99% of malignancies diagnosed in the country are registered [10]. About 1% of the cases are based on death certificate only information.

Available data in the FCR

The Finnish Cancer Registry routinely collects data on demographic information of the patient as well as diagnosis and treatment related data:

- Demographic data
  - Full name
  - PID (for those died before 1967: date of birth)
  - Sex
  - Postal code
  - Municipality of residence in the beginning of the year of diagnosis
- Data on diagnosis of tumour
  - Previous cancer (if any)
  - Primary site of current neoplasm (topography)
  - Date of diagnosis (month, year)
  - Basis of diagnosis
  - Stage at diagnosis (systematically classified as: localised, regional metastases, distant metastases; in later decades also often with TNM information)
  - Behaviour
  - Morphology
- Data on treatment
  - Surgery, radiotherapy, chemotherapy, hormonal therapy, other, none (justification)
- Follow-up data
  - Date and causes of death
  - Date of emigration

Further information on cancer patients such as place of birth, PIDs of relatives, map coordinates of residences, occupation, education, socio-economic position, income etc. are available from Population Register and census files of Statistics Finland, when needed [11]. These high-quality data can be linked to cancer patient data using the PID as the linkage key.

4.1.4 Migration-sensitive cancer research

Compared with other European countries Finland only has a very small number of migrants. Hence, migrant-specific (cancer) research currently does not constitute a relevant topic in science and politics. This is also why studies on cancer among migrants in Finland are almost nonexistent till now. Nevertheless, it can be assumed that migrant-specific research will gain more interest as the number of migrants has been growing continuously over the past years.

There are published results on cancer incidence of one small population group that – like many other evacuees – had to leave their original living area and moved to the current Finnish territory, namely the Skolts, one of the Sami populations. The Sami are one of the most northern arctic indigenous populations whose roots reach back to the oldest known Northern-Fennoscandian population dating back to prehistoric times. There are 10 different Sami languages, 3 of those are spoken in Finland (Inari Sami, North Sami and Skolt Sami). Inari Sami have only lived in Finland, whereas the North Sami share their tradition with Sami from other Nordic countries. Skolts had to leave from the municipality of Petsamo, which now belongs to the Russian Federation, after the Second World War.

In the study by Soininen et al. [3], a cohort of 394 persons with Skolt ethnicity was followed-up for their cancer incidence. On a case-by-case basis the study population was classified as Sami when representing 75-100% of any ethnic group of Sami and also divided into different subgroups of Sami (North Sami, Inari Sami, Skolts).

During the 6,783 person-years of follow-up, the Skolts developed 30 cancer cases, which is slightly more than the expected number of cases (28.8) calculated by multiplying the number of person-years in each sex-age-period stratum by the corresponding average cancer incidence in whole Finland. However, cancer incidence among the Skolts was significantly higher than the incidence among the other Sami ($SIR_{Skolts}/SIR_{otherSami}$ 1.9, 95% CI 1.2–3.0). Skolts had an increased risk of stomach cancer (3.8, 95% CI 1.5-7.8) and to a lesser extent lung cancer (1.7, 95% CI 0.6-3.6), while North Sami and Inari Sami had no increased risk for these cancer types. The $SIR_{Skolts}/SIR_{otherSami}$ for stomach cancer was 6.6 (95% CI 1.8–26.0).

One of the explanations why Skolts are doing worse might be related to their isolated traditional life habits and genetic properties, which are somewhat different from those of other Sami. Soininen and her coworkers [3] describe the low living standard among the Finnish Skolts, who gave up their nomadic lifestyle and moved away from their home district in the late 1940s, as follows: "Fish was eaten dried and sour. Still in 1970 the malnutrition was obvious: Haemoglobin concentrations were low, some had rickets, and children were small and gaunt. There has been a lack of calcium, iron, vitamin C and group B vitamins. In recent decades, the lifestyle of Skolts has changed more than that of other Sami populations. Their traditional livelihood as reindeer herders has declined, and the diet includes less reindeer meat and more white bread, margarine and sugar. It has been postulated that the dietary status of the Skolts corresponded to that of the other Finns 25 years earlier. Taking into account the strongly decreasing trend of stomach cancer incidence in Finland, a 25-year shift backwards in time would correspond to 3- to 4-fold incidence, 30 exactly what we observed among the Skolts."

In Finland, there is an ongoing progress in bringing forward migrant-specific research in other fields, for example in the field of maternal and child health. In this context, Malin and Gissler [12] examined the access to and use of maternity care services as well as birth outcomes by ethnic minority women based on data from the Medical Birth Register (MBR), existing since 1987. Through record linkage between the Population data at Statistics Finland and the MBR by using the women's PID, the authors were able to extend the medical data with information on country of birth, nationality and language as well as family relations. Results have been published along with results of induced abortions [12] and use – not need – of health care services [13].

At times, the conduct of studies on cancer risk among migrants in Finland is being debated, but so far the number of migrants is still considered too small and the follow-up time after immigration too short to obtain valuable and meaningful results. Markedly stronger study settings could be based on combined data of several Nordic countries, such as the census-based five country cohort primarily collected for studies on occupational hazards [14]. The study sources also includes the variable country of birth, and analyses based on that variable are being planned. This is especially relevant in order to determine the role of occupational exposures in cancer aetiology, in particular among migrants whose occupational distribution is different from that of other workers of the Nordic countries.

The Finnish Cancer Registry has a strong tradition of conducting studies on variation in *survival* of cancer patients. A recent study demonstrated that educational level and especially specific knowledge of health-related issues had an impact on survival of most cancer diseases [15]. The same methodology could be well extended to studies on survival differences between cancer patients originating from different countries.

4.1.5 Possibilities to combine cancer cases and denominator population

The routine data collection procedure of the Finnish Cancer Registry does not include variables that allow for the identification of migrants (e.g. country of birth). Therefore, routine tabulations on cancer incidence, mortality or survival among the migrants populations have not been published by the FCR. However, migrant-specific cancer research is possible through data linkage with variables from the National Population Register through linkage on the individual level by the PID that is available in both databases (see paragraph "Cancer risks according to place of birth – a linkage study" below). The FCR introduced that every cancer patient who was alive in 1967 is obliged to have a PID. For persons who died before 1967, a manual (or computer-assisted) record linkage can be done based on names, dates of birth and place of residence [14]. Thus, from the technical perspective, the FCR can easily create a cohort of migrants with data on date of immigration, country of origin and citizenship and calculate epidemiologic measures such as cancer incidence, cancer mortality, and cancer patient survival for such a cohort.

Nevertheless, the need for epidemiological research on cancer risk of the migrants is not seen yet. So even rather negligible aspects impede the implementation of routine analyses on migrant cancer risks: E.g. time consuming permission procedures for data extraction from the National Population Register. Cost of data extraction from the Population Register is not covered in the routine budget of the FCR, i.e., specific project funding would be required. As the number of cancer cases among migrants in Finland is small, it is unlikely that such a study suggestion would successfully compete with other research topics.

Cancer risks according to place of birth – a linkage study

In 2008, the FCR linked its database with the Population Register aiming at studying cancer risks according to place of birth. In this context, it was also possible to identify all cancer patients that were born outside Finland. A simple calculation of the numbers of cancer cases per country of origin (Tab. 4.1.2) reveals that most of the migrant cohorts have significantly less cancers registered in FCR than it would be the case if they had the same incidence of cancer diagnosed and registered in Finland as the averaged population in Finland. Even such rough tabulations made specifically for single cancer types may reveal clues of aetiological differences. For instance, there was a significantly higher incidence of lung cancer among persons born in former Yugoslavia and of cervical cancer among women born in Thailand than among comparable persons born in Finland.

It is known from other countries that the interpretation of cancer risk estimates among migrants is more difficult when the majority has migrated recently [16]. Migrant populations are most likely a self-selected and non-random sample from the population of their countries of origin. Immigrants may often come from very limited sub-areas within the country of origin or from special religions, socio-economic positions, occupations, or ethnic groups. The term "healthy migrant effect" is used to describe the fact that migrants are healthier than the average population in the country of origin [17]. As migration requires a lot of energy and resources the availability of information on the reason for migration (e.g. work, family, refugee, seeking asylum) would support the interpretation of results.

Tab. 4.1.2 *Observed (O) and expected (E)* number of cancer cases diagnosed before 2006 and registered in the Finnish Cancer Registry according to country of birth*

Country of birth	O	O/E**	95% CI**
Soviet Union	1.374	0.85	0.81-0.90
Sweden	386	0.46	0.42-0.51
USA	165	0.51	0.44-0.60
Estonia	120	0.47	0.39-0.56
Germany	93	0.31	0.25-0.38
UK	79	0.54	0.43-0.67
Russian Federation	75	1.00	0.78-1.25
Yugoslavia	72	0.90	0.70-1.13
Canada	49	0.54	0.40-0.72
Irak	40	0.91	0.65-1.24
Vietnam	38	0.78	0.55-1.07
Iran	34	0.83	0.58-1.16
Norway	32	0.44	0.30-0.62
Italy	30	0.63	0.43-0.91
Hungary	28	0.61	0.41-0.88
Poland	27	0.26	0.17-0.38
Somalia	25	0.53	0.34-0.78
Netherlands	23	0.54	0.34-0.81
Denmark	23	0.41	0.26-0.62
Thailand	21	0.64	0.39-0.97
Switzerland	21	0.50	0.31-0.76
China	21	0.38	0.24-0.59
France	21	0.37	0.23-0.57
Afghanistan	18	1.01	0.60-1.60
Turkey	14	0.41	0.23-0.69
India	14	0.38	0.21-0.64
Philippines	11	0.66	0.33-1.19
Australia	11	0.44	0.22-0.78
Japan	11	0.33	0.16-0.59
Israel	10	0.87	0.42-1.59
Spain	10	0.22	0.10-0.40

*   Expected number of cases (E) is based on the proportion of all persons born outside Finland out of all persons with Finnish person identity code; this preliminary data analysis committed for this book was adjusted for calendar period, sex, and year of birth
** Observed to expected ratio (O/E), with its 95% confidence interval (CI).

To reduce the effect of selection bias in migrant studies, researchers should make comparisons between similar groups, immigrants vs. source population in country of origin which is usually impossible. Geographical variation in cancer risk within a *host* country is also considered as a possible source for confounding, given that immigrants are rarely distributed homogeneously in the host country. This can be taken into account in a precise way in Finland where the spatio-temporal variation of cancer incidence is known very detailed [11]. Socio-economic position is known to be a strong determinant of cancer in Finland as in other countries in terms of both cancer incidence [18-21] and survival [15, 22]. It is often clear from census data that migrants are overrepresented in specific occupational categories and are atypical of the general population in their socio-economic profile. One should therefore use socioeconomic position or occupation–specific reference rates in risk calculations. This is in principle possible in the Nordic countries by using census files [14]. Migrant populations who have been living long enough in Finland and have their occupation, education and socio-economic position registered in the census database. These variables are also recorded in an accurate way comparable to those recorded for non-migrant populations.

A further bias might result from inequalities in access to healthcare facilities for immigrants compared with the native population, and from re-migration related to cancer symptoms. The problem arises if immigrants return to their country of origin due to critical status of their health and the probability of passing away there. If the dates of re-migration are not registered, the overcoverage in the population statistics leads to overestimation of person-years at risk and, and subsequently to further underestimation of the incidence of the health outcome under study. There are no estimates of this error for Finnish migrants but in Sweden, with quite similar population registration procedure, the overcoverage is estimated to range from 4 to 8% for non-Nordic immigrants [23]. No overcoverage has been observed for immigrants from Nordic countries because since 1969 Nordic countries have coordinated their population changes with each other.

4.1.6 Conclusions

So far, there has been almost no research on cancer in migrants in Finland. However, migrant-specific analyses would be feasible by linkage procedures. The PID is a good instrument to conduct migrant-specific research. Its feasibility and the data accuracy have successfully been tested and carried out in routine plausibility checks.

The number of migrants coming to Finland has been growing in the past years, comprising merely a small but heterogeneous population. Looking at the demographic changes, a further increase of migrants from other EU and non EU-countries to Finland is to be expected. As we know from other European countries, migrants tend to have other health risks and behaviours than the autochthonous population, which also applies to cancer risks and cancer related risk factors, e.g. lifestyle. This development elucidates the relevance of this topic in future research in Finland as well as its implications for politics and practice. In other fields (related to younger age strata than cancer), e.g. maternal and child health, Finland has already made good progress in terms of migrant-specific and migrant-sensitive research. These are essential steps in understanding strengths and pitfalls in register-based information on migrants and offer important implications for the migrant cancer research when the time for such studies will be mature.

Acknowledgement

The authors are grateful to Professors Timo Hakulinen (Finnish Cancer Registry) and Mika Gissler (THL National Institute for Health and Welfare, Finland) for their valuable and constructive advice in approving the Finnish country report in its final form.

References

1. Population Structure 2009. 2010 19.08.2010]; Available from: www.stat.fi/til/vaerak/2009/vaerak_2009_2010-03-19_en.pdf.
2. Population density. 2010 19.08.2010]; Available from: http://www.stat.fi/tup/verkkokoulu/data/vt/05/06/index_en.html.
3. Soininen, L., S. Jarvinen, and E. Pukkala, Cancer incidence among Sami in Northern Finland, 1979-1998. Int J Cancer, 2002. 100(3): p. 342-6.
4. Migration 2008. 2009, Statistics Finland.
5. Statistics Finland's PX-Web databases. 2010, Statistics Finland
6. Population Information System. 2006; Available from: http://www.vrk.fi/vrk/home.nsf/www/population
7. Järvelin, J., Health Care Systems in Transition. Finland. 2002, European Observatory on Health Care Systems.
8. Teperi, J., et al., The Finnish Health Care System. A Value-Based Perspective, in Sitra Report, E. Prima, Editor. 2009: Helsinki.
9. FKI, Cancer incidence in Finland 2008. 2010, Finnish Cancer Registry - Institute for Statistical and Epidemiological Cancer Research
10. Teppo, L., E. Pukkala, and M. Lehtonen, Data quality and quality control of a population-based cancer registry. Experience in Finland. Acta Oncologica, 1994. 33(4): p. 365-9.
11. Pukkala, E. and T. Patama, Small-area based map animations of cancer incidence in the Finland, 1953-2008. 2010, Finnish Cancer Registry.
12. Malin, M. and M. Gissler, Induced abortions among immigrant women in Finland. Finnish Journal of Ethnicity and Migration, 2008. 3: p. 2-12.

13. Gissler, M., M. Malin, and P. Matveinen. Terveydenhuollon palvelut ja sosiaalihuollon laitospalvelut. Julkaisussa: Maahanmuuttajat ja julkiset palvelut. 2006; Available from: http://www.mol.fi/mol/fi/99_pdf/fi/06_tyoministerio/06_julkaisut/06_tutkimus/tpt296.pdf.

14. Pukkala, E., et al., Occupation and cancer - follow-up of 15 million people in five Nordic countries. Acta Oncologica, 2009. 48(5): p. 646-790.

15. Pokhrel, A., et al., Education, survival and avoidable deaths in cancer patients in Finland. Br J Cancer, 2010. 103(7): p. 1109-14.

16. Beiki, O., Cancer and Migration: Epidemiological studies on relationship between country of birth, socio-economic position and cancer. 2010, Karolinska Intitutet: Stockholm.

17. Marmot, M.G., A.M. Adelstein, and L. Bulusu, Lessons from the study of immigrant mortality. Lancet, 1984. 1(8392): p. 1455-7.

18. Pukkala, E., Cancer risk by social class and occupation. A survey of 109,000 cancer cases among Finns of working age. Contributions to Epidemiology and Biostatistics, 1995. 7.

19. Pukkala, E. and E. Weiderpass, Time trends in socio-economic differences in incidence rates of cancers of the breast and female genital organs (Finland, 1971-1995). Int J Cancer, 1999. 81(1): p. 56-61.

20. Pukkala, E. and E. Weiderpass, Socio-economic differences in incidence rates of cancers of the male genital organs in Finland, 1971-95. Int J Cancer, 2002. 102(6): p. 643-8.

21. Weiderpass, E. and E. Pukkala, Time trends in socioeconomic differences in incidence rates of cancers of gastro-intestinal tract in Finland. BMC Gastroenterol, 2006. 6: p. 41.

22. Auvinen, A., S. Karjalainen, and E. Pukkala, Social class and cancer patient survival in Finland. Am J Epidemiol, 1995. 142(10): p. 1089-102.

23. Qvist, J., Problems of coverage in the register of total population (RTB). Estimation of overcoverage with an indirect method. 1999, Statistics Sweden: Örebro, Sweden.

4.2 Germany

Jacob Spallek^{1,2}, Stefan Hentschel^3

1   Bielefeld University, Department of Epidemiology and International Public Health, Germany
2   University of Bremen, Bremen Institute for Prevention Research and Social Medicine, Germany
3   Hamburgisches Krebsregister, Hamburg, Germany

4.2.1 General information about Germany

Germany has a total area of 357,112 km² and a population of 81.76 million in 2010. The population density is with 229 inhabitants per km² high. The country is organized in a federal system and has 16 federal states *(Bundesländer)*.

Immigrant Population in Germany

Germany has the largest immigrant population in Europe. Today a proportion of about 20% of the population living in Germany has a migrant background. Based on the Mikrozensus – a census of the Federal Statistical Office of Germany – more than 15 million persons residing in Germany are migrants of first or second generation (see tab. 4.2.1).

Tab. 4.2.1:   *Population with migrant background, foreign population and number of naturalisations in Germany [1]*

	2007	2008	2009
	in 1,000		
Population (Mikrozensus)	82,257	82,135	81,904
Persons with migrant background (Mikrozensus)	15,411	15,566	15,703
Foreign population (Ausländerzentralregister)	6,745	6,728	6,695
Number of naturalisations (Einbürgerungsstatistik)	113	94	96

Because of Germany's central location in Europe it has always been both a thoroughfare and an immigration country. In addition to a large intake of refugees after the Second World War, two major immigration movements occurred since the 1950s [2].

1. In the 1960s, Germany started recruiting "guest workers". The majority of these workers came from southern and east-southern European countries (Portugal, Spain, Italy, Yugoslavia, Greece and Turkey) and although originally planned to be temporary, many of them chose to reside in Germany permanently.

2. The immigration of ethnic Germans known as "Spät-Aussiedler" (resettlers, in contrast to the first migration directly after the Second World War). To date more than 4 million "Spät-Aussiedler" have migrated to Germany,

principally from the former Soviet Union. Of these, about 2.5 million have come since the fall of the Iron Curtain in 1989. These resettlers are predominantly the descendants of Germans who migrated to East Europe in the 17th and 18th century.

The largest group of immigrants with approximately 4 million persons is the group of these so called resettlers, who have mostly obtained German citizenship directly after migration, or even before. The second largest group are immigrants from Turkey. About 1.71 million (25%) of the 6.6 million foreigners in Germany are of Turkish nationality. Roughly a further 750,000 Turks have become naturalized citizens since the 1990s, altogether making up more than 2.5 million persons and close to 3% of the entire German population (Federal Statistical Office 2008). The next largest groups of foreigners are Italian (>500,000), Serbian/Republic of Yugoslavian (<500,000), Polish (>320,000) and Croatian (<230,000) [3]. The number of so called illegal immigrants in Germany is unknown. Tentative appraisals give numbers between 500,000 and 1,000,000.

Availability of information on ethnicity in German routine health data

In Germany there is still a paucity of data on the health situation of migrants. The major problem, among others, is the unavailability of information on ethnicity or migrant background in health data. Data protection laws are, partly as a result of the persecution of ethnic minorities in German history, very strict with regard to information on race or ethnicity. Some health data include information on citizenship, but exclude the group of naturalized migrants. They also do not take dual citizenships into account, thus excluding the majority of the population with migrant backgrounds. Over the past years the situation has improved and more routine data (e.g. the Mikrozensus) or surveys (e.g. the Child and Youth Health Survey KIGGS; www.kiggs.de) collect anonymous and voluntarily elaborated data on ethnicity/migrant background/country of birth.

4.2.2 The German Health Care system

Germany has the oldest universal health care system in Europe, originating from the social legislation of Otto von Bismarck in 1883. Currently about 85% of the population are mandatory members of the basic health insurance plan (Gesetzliche Krankenversicherung, GKV) that provides a standard routine level of health care. The remainder, mostly high income employees or freelancers who are not mandatory members of the GKV, are members of private health insurance companies (Private Krankenversicherung, PKV) which offer some additional benefits.

The GKV covers all costs of necessary medical treatment and rehabilitation. GKV – and PKV – are struggling with the increasing costs of medical treatment and the changing demography. In the GKV, co-payments for drugs and medically not justified treatments were introduced in the 1980s in an attempt to prevent over-utilization. The health-care reform law that took effect on January 1, 2004, aimed at reducing health insurance costs. Costs were to be stabilized by introducing more competition into the health-care system and requiring higher co-payments, e.g. for drugs, by the insured. Nevertheless the costs and monthly rates which are co-financed by employer and employee (about 15% of the monthly gross income) are increasing. Health care expenditures in Germany amount to about 11% of GDP, comparable to other western European nations, but substantially less than spent by the U.S. (nearly 16% of GDP) [4].

Germany has a very good working health care system that covers the huge majority of the German population. The country is ranking 30th in the world in life expectancy (78 years for men), and has a very low infant mortality rate (4.7 per 1,000 live births).

Besides the health insurance system, Germany has two other health benefit systems: the accident insurance and the long-term care insurance. Insurance for working accidents (Arbeitsunfallversicherung) is paid by the employer and basically covers all risks for commuting to and from work, and at the workplace. Long-term nursing care (Pflegeversicherung) is equally paid for by the employer and the employee and covers cases in which a person is not able to manage his or her daily routine due to illness (provision of food, cleaning of apartment, personal hygiene, etc.).

4.2.3 Cancer registration in Germany

In Germany, cancer registration for adults is organized under the responsibility of the federal states. The federal state of Hamburg has one of the oldest cancer registries in the world which has been operating since the late 1920s. In other federal states cancer registration started later: 1967 in the Saarland and 1986 in Münster, a region of the federal state North Rhine-Westfalia. In the former so called German Democratic Republik (GDR), cancer registration was established in the 1950s. As a consequence of a new cancer registration law (Krebsregistergesetz KRG), cancer registries were established in most federal states from 1995-1999. In 2010, the federal cancer registration law (Bundeskrebsregistergesetz BKRG) stipulating that all federal states should have their own cancer registration law and establish cancer registration was enacted (see fig. 4.2.1). At present, 14 federal states have implemented cancer registration that fits international standards in terms of data quality, completeness and standardization.

All cancer registries are organized under the Association of Population-based Cancer Registries in Germany (GEKID e.V., see www.gekid.de). In cooperation with the Robert Koch-Institut (Federal German Health Authority), this association publishes a brochure with data on cancer in Germany every two years. The brochure includes data from all cancer registries and estimations about completeness.

Fig. 4.2.1: *Federal states with cancer registration in Germany*

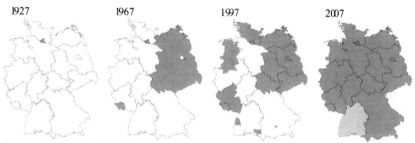

Source: http://www.gekid.de.

A special situation exists for childhood cancers in Germany. The registration of cancer cases among children younger than 18 years is additionally organized nationwide via therapy studies and represented by the German Childhood Cancer Registry located in Mainz.

Available data in the cancer registries

The German population-based cancer registries routinely collect data on demographic information, on tumours and on patient survival.

Generally this includes:

- Demographic data:
  - first name and surname (as well as change of name)
  - sex
  - date of birth (date, month, year)
  - place of residence (address, postal code)
- Data on diagnosis of tumour:
  - source of information
  - tumour site and type
  - date of diagnosis
  - basis and certainty of the diagnosis
  - method of first detection
  - topography and laterality, the localisation of the tumour
  - morphology, tissue typing
  - TNM for some cancers
  - tumour histology

- Treatment data:
  - type of treatment (surgery, radiotherapy, chemotherapy, other therapy)
- Follow-up data:
  - cause of death
  - date of death

4.2.4 Migration-sensitive cancer research

Some cancer registries collect data on nationality based on citizenship or assignment by the reporting person (usually the treating doctor). As information on nationality is generally irrelevant with respect to diagnosis and treatment, the quality of these data remains limited in terms of validity and completeness. Hence – as in most German health data bases – routine analyses in German cancer registries are not migrant sensitive or migrant specific.

Data linkage procedures are impossible because no other complete and population based data containing information on migrant background or ethnicity are available. At federal state level only data with citizenship are available. These data are however of limited usefulness for migrant health research as it is not possible to identify naturalized migrants

As a consequence, research on cancer among migrants in Germany had to pursue alternative ways to identify cancer cases in registry data (cancer registries or death registries) and to estimate the number of migrants using the same method in the corresponding denominator population:

(1) a name based approach to identify persons with Turkish names [5-6]
(2) data linkage procedures to combine data from death registries or cancer registries with data on place of residence of German resettlers (Spät-Aussiedler) [7].

Several research projects have been conducted based on these approaches:
1. Cancer incidence and survival among Turkish children in Germany

In an analysis of the data of the German Childhood Cancer Registry including all cancer cases in Germany from 1980-2005, Spallek et al. [6] used a name based approach to identify the cases with Turkish names. An estimation of the denominator population – meaning all children with Turkish names in Germany – was not possible. Therefore a case only analysis using the measure of proportional cancer incidence ratios was performed. In this analysis children with Turkish names had more often acute non-lymphocytic leukaemia, Hodgkin's Disease and Non-Hodgkin/Burkitt lymphoma than non Turkish children. Age, sex and period of diagnosis did not influence the distribution of diagnoses [8]. Based on this study, Spix et al. [9] analysed the survival of cases with Turkish names and without Turkish names using the Kaplan-Meier method and log rank-test. No differences, overall and age- or sex-specific, in 5-year survival probability for all cancers were found.

2. Cancer incidence of Turkish persons in Hamburg

In this study Spallek et al. [10] were able to identify Turkish persons based on the name-based approach in the Cancer Registry Hamburg and in the corresponding population under risk (denominator), and calculated sex- and age-specific cancer incidence rates for Turkish and Non-Turkish persons in Hamburg from 1990-2005.

Cancer of the respiratory organs was diagnosed less frequently among Turkish men in older birth cohorts but with higher frequency in the younger birth cohorts. The incidence of malignant neoplasms of lymphoid, haematopoietic and related tissues was slightly higher in most male Turkish men birth cohorts than in non-Turkish birth cohorts. Among women, incidence rates for Turkish women were lower than for non-Turkish women for cancer of the respiratory system, skin cancer and cancer of genital organs. Also, breast cancer incidence rates of Turkish women were lower than for non-Turkish women, especially in older birth cohorts. Incidence rate ratios of neoplasms of lymphoid, haematopoietic and related tissues were low in the 1931 to <1941 cohort, but increased in younger birth cohorts.

3. Cancer mortality of German resettlers in North Rhine-Westfalia (Spät-Aussiedler)

Kyobutungi et al. [11] and Becher et al. [12] compared the cancer mortality of German resettlers to that of the general population in the federal state North Rhine-Westfalia (Nordrhein-Westfalen) using a data linkage approach [7]. The overall cancer mortality of the resettlers was lower than that of the general population. Cancer mortality for lung cancer, cancer of the stomach and – in the analyses of Becher et al. for liver cancer –was higher for male resettlers. Prostate mortality was lower among the male resettlers. Compared to the general population, female resettlers had a higher cancer mortality for stomach cancer and a lower mortality for breast cancer. Ronellenfitsch et al. [13] reanalysed the same study cohort with the aim to gain possible explanations of the differences in stomach cancer mortality that are attributable to early life exposures to infections and other hygiene conditions.

4. Cancer mortality and incidence in German resettlers in North Rhine-Westfalia and Saarland

Winkler et al. [14] combined the results of the North Rhine-Westfalian resettler cohort with new data based on a linkage of the cancer registry of the Saarland with data about residence of resettlers in the Saarland. They found higher cancer incidences of the liver and stomach among male and female resettlers, and a higher lung cancer incidence among male resettlers. These were comparable to the higher cancer mortality among the same cancer sites found in the previous studies. New findings were a higher cancer incidence and mortality for brain tumours among male resettlers and a higher leukaemia incidence among both male and female resettlers.

4.2.5 Possibilities to combine cancer cases and denominator population

In Germany, ethnicity is currently only recorded accurately in the *Mikrozensus*. These data are useful to estimate the number and some socio-demographic information on migrants in Germany. Information on immigrant background from *Mikrozensus* has not been linked to registry data at the moment because of data protection restrictions and methodological problems (anonymisation, sampling).

Since data on migrant background/ethnicity do not exist in the regional cancer registries and no general population data including these information are available for linkage procedures, migration-sensitive cancer research in Germany is restricted to individual efforts for analysing data about specific migrant groups (e.g. Turkish or Resettlers) in specific cancer registries.

There are plans to continue the research as described in the studies above and – besides further analyses of cancer risks – to conduct analyses on breast cancer screening uptake, stage distribution, use of treatment and survival in the future.

4.2.6 Conclusion

Up to now several studies have been performed to analyse cancer risks and survival of migrants in Germany. There are some main aspects characterizing the situation. First, there is wariness concerning the collection of personal data, e.g. about ethnicity, in Germany, partly caused by the specific German history, resulting in strict data protection laws. Second, as the issue of nationality resp. ethnicity or migration background does not concern the medical care, one cannot expect to get valid information on that subject from medical records. In addition, there is limited scientific attention to the topic of migrant specific health which is hindering efforts to collect these data routinely and nationwide in a sustainable way.

It is possible that in the future the statistical offices will introduce better population based data on persons with migrant backgrounds, and that with these new data new possibilities for data linkage procedures will emerge.

Further steps/ Future prospects

In the near future research on cancer in migrants will continue with individual studies on risk and survival of specific migrant groups in specific areas.

However, with increasing awareness of the diversity of the German population, it is anticipated that more data will contain information on ethnicity/migrant background. This will hopefully lead to more possibilities for data linkage procedures, and in the end, to the inclusion of a migrant perspective in routine analyses of cancer data in Germany.

References

1. Destatis. Migration und Integration. 2010; Available from: http://www.destatis.de/jet speed/portal/cms/Sites/destatis/Internet/DE/Navigation/Statistiken/Bevoelkerung/Migrati onIntegration/MigrationIntegration.psml

2. Razum, O., Migration und Gesundheit – Schwerpunktbericht der Gesundheitsberichterstattung des Bundes, RKI, Editor. 2008, Robert Koch-Institut: Berlin.

3. Destatis, Ausländische Bevölkerung 2009, Federal Statistical Office of Germany: Wiesbaden.

4. Borger, C., et al., Health spending projections through 2015: Changes on the horizon. Health Affairs, 2006: p. W61-W73.

5. Razum, O., H. Zeeb, and S. Akgun, How useful is a name-based algorithm in health research among Turkish migrants in Germany? Tropical medicine & international health: TM & IH, 2001. 6(8): p. 654-61.

6. Spallek, J., et al., [Name-based identification of cases of Turkish origin in the childhood cancer registry in Mainz]. Gesundheitswesen, 2006. 68(10): p. 643-9.

7. Ronellenfitsch, U., et al., Large-scale, population-based epidemiological studies with record linkage can be done in Germany. European Journal of Epidemiology, 2004. 19(12): p. 1073-1074.

8. Spallek, J., et al., Cancer patterns among children of Turkish descent in Germany: a study at the German Childhood Cancer Registry. BMC Public Health, 2008. 8: p. 152.

9. Spix, C., et al., Cancer survival among children of Turkish descent in Germany 1980-2005: a registry-based analysis. BMC Cancer, 2008. 8: p. 355.

10. Spallek, J., et al., Cancer incidence rate ratios of Turkish immigrants in Hamburg, Germany: A registry based study. Cancer epidemiology, 2009. 33(6): p. 413-8.

11. Kyobutungi, C., et al., Mortality from cancer among ethnic German immigrants from the Former Soviet Union, in Germany. Eur J Cancer, 2006. 42(15): p. 2577-84.

12. Becher, H., et al., Mortalität von Aussiedlern aus der ehemaligen SU. Ergebnisse einer Kohortenstudie. Deutsches Ärzteblatt 104, 2007. 104: p. A1655-A1661.

13. Ronellenfitsch, U., et al., *Stomach cancer mortality in two large cohorts of migrants from the Former Soviet Union to Israel and Germany: are there implications for prevention?* Eur J Gastroenterol Hepatol, 2009. 21(4): p. 409-16.

14. Winkler, V., et al., *Cancer profile of migrants from the Former Soviet Union in Germany: incidence and mortality.* Cancer Causes Control, 2009.

4.3 The Netherlands

Anna Reeske[1], Sabine Siesling[2], Jacob Spallek[1,3],
Melina Arnold[3], Otto Visser[4]

1   University of Bremen, Bremen Institute for Prevention Research and Social Medicine,
     Germany
2   Integraal Kankercentrum Nederland (IKNL), locations Groningen and Enschede, The
     Netherlands
3   Bielefeld University, Department for Epidemiology and International Public Health,
     Germany
4   Integraal Kankercentrum Nederland (IKNL), location Amsterdam, The Netherlands

4.3.1 General information about The Netherlands

The Netherlands consist of 12 provinces and 418 municipalities as well as territories in the Caribbean (former colonies). The Netherlands has a total area of 33,883 km² and with a population of more than 16 million, it represents the 28th most densely populated country in the world (of 400.4 inhabitants per square kilometre). The majority of the population lives in the *randstad,* a conurbation of the four largest cities and its surroundings in the West of the Netherlands: Amsterdam, Rotterdam, The Hague and Utrecht (see fig. 4.3.1). The official language is Dutch, although there are several dialects and recognised regional languages such as Low Saxon, Limburgish, Frisian and Papiamento (spoken by some people from the Caribbean islands).

Population

In 2010, the Netherlands have a population size of 16.6 million. The origin of the population is diverse, with about 13.2 million natives and 3.4 million people with a foreign background (first or second generation), corresponding to 20.3% of the population or every fifth citizen. Of all persons with a foreign background, 55.3% (1.9 million) come from non-western countries, whereas 44.7% (1.4 million) come from western countries. The largest immigrant groups come from Turkey (11.4% of all persons with foreign background), Indonesia (11.4%), Germany (11.3%), Morocco (10.4%), Suriname (10.2%), and the Netherlands Antilles and Aruba (4.1%) [1].

Table 4.3.1 shows the absolute numbers and proportions of persons with a foreign background residing in the Netherlands. A person with a background of first degree (first generation) is defined as born abroad with at least one parent born abroad. A person with a background of second degree (second generation) is accordingly defined as born in the Netherlands with at least one parents born abroad.

Fig. 4.3.1:   *Population density in the Netherlands, 2010*

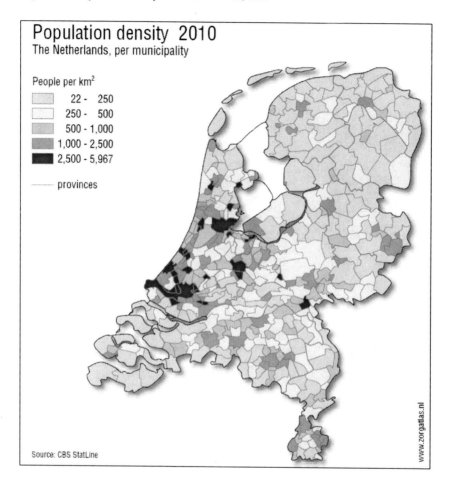

Population Registration in the Netherlands

The Netherlands consist of more than 400 municipalities that collect all events such as birth, death and migration. All municipalities are part of a national electronic network that enables the exchange of data. Statistics Netherlands (*Centraal Bureau voor de Statistiek* – CBS) is also part of the network and brings together the population data. So it is possible to describe and analyse the population data by country of origin for the whole of the Netherlands.

Availability of information on migration background

Information on country of birth, parental country of birth and nationality are available in nearly all data bases of the municipalities.

Tab. 4.3.2: Population according to origin and generation, both sexes combined, 2009 [1]

Origin	Total	First generation	%	Second generation	%
Native (autochtonous)	13,198,081				
Foreign (allochthonous)	3,287,706	1,661,505	50,5	1,626,201	49,5
Western*	1,478,396	627,311	42,4	851,085	57,6
Non-Western**	1,809,310	1,034,194	57,2	775,116	42,8
Morocco	341,528	166,774	48,8	174,754	51,2
Netherlands Antilles/Aruba	134,774	79,785	59,2	54,989	40,8
Suriname	338,678	184,961	54,6	153,717	45,4
Turkey	378,330	195,375	51,6	182,955	48,4
Indonesia	384,497	121,289	31,5	263,208	68,5

*   Europe (except Turkey), North-America, Oceania, Indonesia and Japan
** Africa, Latin-America and Asia (except Japan and Indonesia)

4.3.2 The Dutch healthcare system

In the Netherlands, it is mandatory for all legal residents and those paying income tax to purchase health insurance at least at a basic level (*basisverzekering*) since the new Health Insurance Act in 2006. However, approximately 1.5% of the population is estimated to be uninsured. In general, coverage is exclusively provided by private health insurers and regulated under private law. The insured may choose their insurer freely and insurers are obliged to accept every applicant in their area of activity. Thus, the health insurance market is highly regulated by competition. Risk equalisation is carried out in order to prevent risk selection by insurers.

The basic insurance covers medical care (including care by general practitioners (GPs), hospitals and midwives), hospitalisation, dental care, medical aids, medicines, maternity care, ambulance and patient transport services and specific paramedical care. Furthermore, every citizen is covered by the statutory Exceptional Medical Expenses Act (AWBZ), comprising a wide range of chronic and mental health care services such as home care and care in nursing homes. Complementary private health insurance for services outside of the standard benefit package is purchased by many citizens. [2]

In 2008, the Dutch healthcare system was rated the best in Europe and was even considered as a model for the US healthcare reform.

4.3.3 Cancer registration in the Netherlands

The Netherlands Cancer Registry

Cancer registration has a long tradition in the Netherlands, but in 1989 the Netherlands Cancer Registry (NCR) was founded, collecting population-based data on the national level. Data for the national registry are collected by registration clerks in two comprehensive cancer centres (CCCs), covering the Netherlands. More than 300 employees work in these centres and about 400 consultants are actively involved. CCCs are independent, private institutions, and all hospitals, radiological centres and pathology labs are affiliated to one of the centres [3].

The nation-wide Dutch pathology laboratory network and registry for histopathology and cytopathology, regularly submits reports of all diagnosed malignancies to the cancer registry. The national hospital discharge databank, receiving discharge diagnoses of admitted patients from all Dutch hospitals, complete case ascertainment. After notification, trained registry personnel collect data on diagnosis, staging and treatment from the medical records, including pathology and surgery reports from the patient files, using the registration and coding manual of NCR. Nation-wide incidence and mortality data for cancer are published annually on the ikcnet-website [3].

Completeness and accuracy of data

Regarding the completeness of Dutch cancer registry data, one regional analysis, using a capture-recapture approach, resulted in an estimation of 98.3% [4]. Furthermore, a study in Limburg, suggests a completeness of 96.2% [5].

Available data in the cancer registry

The NCR is a tumour registry, meaning that for certain patients, more than one tumour can appear in the registry. Variables routinely collected in the NCR are based on coding systems of the World Health Organisation (WHO) and the International Association of Cancer Registries (IACR) in order to facilitate international comparisons. The topography and morphology are coded using the International Classification of Diseases for Oncology (ICD-O). The stage of the tumour at diagnosis is determined according to the TNM classification [3].

The following variables are part of the routine data collection:

- Demographic data:
  - patient identification code
  - date of birth
  - sex

- postal code at diagnosis
- place/country of birth
- Hospital data:
  - hospital of diagnosis
- Data on the diagnosis:
  - tumour serial number (indicating the order if more than one tumour is found in a patient)
  - date of incidence (date of diagnosis)
  - basis of the diagnosis
  - topography and laterality (localisation of primary tumour)
  - morphology, tissue typing
  - number of examined/positive lymph nodes
  - cTNM, pTNM
  - residual disease after surgery
  - site-specific variables (such as prognostic scores, tumour markers)

- Treatment data:
  - type of treatment
  - start of treatment
  - hospital of treatment
- Follow-up data:
  - status of patient (indicates if the patient is still alive)
  - date of death/date of last contact

4.3.4 Migration-sensitive cancer research

During the past year, several studies analysing cancer among immigrants by linking data of the cancer registry to population data have been conducted in the Netherlands. Data linkage is possible on the basis of several variables e.g. name or date of birth. In this section, methods and findings of selected studies are presented.

Breast and stomach cancer incidence and survival in migrants in the Netherlands 1996-2006 [6]

Arnold and colleagues (2010), for the first time, analysed cancer incidence and survival in the largest migrant groups using data on the national level. Cancer cases were obtained from the NCR, population data from Statistics Netherlands.

Tab. 4.3.3: Standardised Incidence Ratios (SIR) for males and females according to country of birth (1996-2006) * [6]

		Native Dutch	Antilles/ Aruba			Indonesia			Morocco			Suriname			Turkey		
		SIR	N	SIR	95% CI	N	SIR	95% CI	N	SIR	95% CI	N	SIR	95% CI	N	SIR	95% CI
Breast Cancer	F	1.0 (Ref)	239	**0.5**	0.4 0.6	1,513	**0.6**	0.5 0.6	193	**0.3**	0.2 0.3	590	**0.4**	0.4 0.4	266	**0.3**	0.2 0.3
Stomach Cancer	F	1.0 (Ref)	25	1.3	0.9 1.9	79	**0.4**	0.3 0.5	34	1.3	0.9 1.8	71	1.0	0.8 1.3	56	**1.5**	1.2 2.0
	M	1.0 (Ref)	39	1.3	0.9 1.8	128	**0.4**	0.3 0.4	73	0.8	0.6 1.0	115	1.0	0.9 1.3	130	**1.4**	1.2 1.7
Cardia	F	1.0 (Ref)	4	1.1	0.4 2.9	19	**0.5**	0.3 0.8	3	0.6	0.2 1.9	12	1.0	0.5 1.7	4	0.6	0.2 1.5
	M	1.0 (Ref)	6	**0.5**	0.2 1.2	58	**0.5**	0.4 0.7	14	**0.4**	0.3 0.7	13	**0.3**	0.2 0.6	19	**0.6**	0.4 0.9
Non-cardia	F	1.0 (Ref)	21	1.3	0.9 2.1	60	**0.4**	0.3 0.5	31	**1.5**	1.0 2.1	59	1.1	0.8 1.4	52	**1.7**	1.3 2.3
	M	1.0 (Ref)	33	**1.8**	1.2 2.5	70	**0.3**	0.2 0.4	59	1.0	0.8 1.3	102	**1.4**	1.2 1.7	111	**1.9**	1.6 2.3

* Bold numbers are significant at 0.05 level; F=Females; M=Males.

Calculating standardized incidence ratios (SIR) for breast and stomach cancer, they found significantly lower breast cancer risks but significantly elevated risks of noncardia stomach cancer in all migrant groups in comparison to Dutch natives (see tab. 4.3.4). Furthermore, 5yr relative survival rates (RSR) of breast cancer were poorer in all migrants, whereas 1yr relative survival of stomach cancer was better in all migrant groups compared to Dutch natives.

Cancer risk in first generation migrants in North-Holland/Flevoland, 1995-2004 [7]

Visser and Van Leeuwen (2007) analysed cancer risks in first generation migrants in North-Holland/Flevoland in 1995-2004. All primary invasive cancers diagnosed among first generation migrants living in North-Holland and Flevoland for the period 1995-2004 were used. The authors linked cancer cases with annual population data from Statistics Netherlands by name and date of birth. First generation immigrants were defined as residents that were born outside the Netherlands.

In this study 106,415 cases were included in the analysis. Within this sample nearly 9% were identified as first generation migrants. 5.3% of the persons born abroad were from western countries (mainly from Indonesia and Germany) and 3.5% from non-western countries (mainly from Suriname, Turkey, Morocco and The Netherlands Antilles).

In comparison to the population born in the Netherlands, almost all countries had a significantly decreased cancer risk, except for Germany, the UK, Belgium and Italy. The lowest cancer risks were observed in migrants from Turkey, Morocco and sub-Sahara Africa (fig. 4.3.3).

SIRs were also calculated for different cancer sites. The highest SIRs were found for cancer of the nasopharynx: among migrants from China (SIR=51), Morocco (SIR=22), Turkey (SIR=8), sub-Sahara Africa (SIR=6), Surinam (SIR=4.6) and Indonesia (SIR=1.2). There were also exceptionally high SIRs for liver cancer (migrants from China (SIR=14), sub-Sahara Africa (SIR=6), Turkey (SIR=4.6), Surinam (SIR=3.3)), gallbladder (migrants from Netherlands Antilles (SIR=6.5)), cervix uteri (migrants from Surinam (SIR=1.7), Morocco (SIR=1.6)), thyroid gland (migrants from Turkey (SIR=2.9), Morocco (SIR=2.3)) and Kaposi's sarcoma (migrants from EU 14 (SIR=6.8), Netherlands Antilles (SIR=5.5), sub-Sahara Africa (SIR=5.4)).

Furthermore, the study showed that cancer sites that are more likely to be found in the native population of the Netherlands (like in most Western countries), such as cancer of the breast, colorectum, lung and prostate gland were generally low in migrants from non-western countries, except for prostate cancer among men born in Suriname (SIR=1.5) and lung cancer among men born in Turkey (SIR=1.2, although not statistically significant). The risks for Hodgkin's lymphoma and mature T/NK-cell neoplasms were increased among migrants, but in general the risks for haematological malignancies were comparable with the risks in the population born in the Netherlands.

Fig. 4.3.3: *Standardised incidence ratio (SIR) with 95% confidence intervals of all cancers combined according to country of birth [7]*

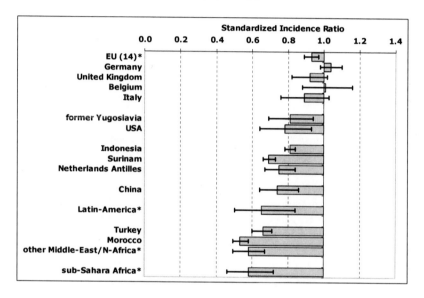

Cancer mortality rates among first and second generation migrants in the Netherlands [8]

Stirbu and colleagues (2006) analysed differences in cancer mortality rates among first and second generation migrants from Turkey, Morocco, Surinam, the Netherlands Antilles and Aruba and the native Dutch population for the period 1995-2000. They linked data from the national cause of death registry to data of the municipal population registers by personal identification numbers. The different migrant groups were defined by country of birth and were assigned as non-native if the person itself or one of the parents was born abroad.

Legal residents entered the study throughout the study period, so the study analysis is based on person years (open cohort design).

The overall cancer mortality rate was lower among all migrant groups (RR varied between 0.40 for Moroccans and 0.78 for Antilleans/Arubans) compared to the rate of the native Dutch population (RR=0.55). For a large number of cancers, migrants had a more than 50% lower risk of death, e.g. for lung cancer

(RR=0.33), colorectal cancer (RR=0.54), and breast cancer (RR=0.53). Elevated risk were found for liver cancer among migrants from Turkey and Suriname (RR above 2.2) and for stomach cancer among Antilleans/Arubans (RR=2.06) as well as migrants from Turkey and Suriname (but not statistically significant).

Mortality rates for all cancers were higher among second generation migrants (those who were younger and had a longer duration of stay), but for most cancer sites the mortality rates among the second generation was lower compared with the native Dutch population.

As far as first generation migrants were concerned, the results of this mortality study were generally consistent with the results of the incidence study of Visser and van Leeuwen [7].

Ethnic inequalities in age- and cause-specific mortality in The Netherlands [9]

Bos et and colleagues analysed ethnic inequalities in age- and cause-specific mortality between migrants from non-Western countries and the native Dutch population for the time period 1995-2000. Migrants were defined as people who themselves or one of the parents were born in Turkey, Morocco, Surinam or the Dutch Antilles/Aruba. As it has been done in the study of Stirbu and colleagues, data from the national cause of death registry have been linked to data of the municipal population registers by personal identification numbers. The cancer specific mortality was analysed based on all malignancies, but especially for lung and stomach cancer as well as breast cancer among females.

Migrants from Turkey, Surinam and Antilles/Aruba had in general a higher risk of dying (about 25%) than the native Dutch population. Only the Moroccans had a RR of 0.85. Among females, the risk was only statistically significant for migrants from Suriname (RR=1.10).

For all cancer combined, the mortality rate ratios (MRR) were low for all migrant groups. Rates for lung cancer were also surprisingly low for all groups and breast cancer among females was also found to be low. In contrast, mortality rate ratios for stomach cancer were high for all migrant groups except for Moroccans, but without statistical significance.

The presented studies show that it is possible to conduct migrant specific cancer research in the Netherlands. Nevertheless, all studies have been done by data linkage procedures. The main problem of these procedures is that they demand a lot of time and budget so they cannot be done routinely.

Nevertheless, the interest in this topic is large, mainly ascribed to an increasing ethnic diversity of the Dutch population. In addition to the above mentioned studies, the *Signaleringscommissie Kanker van KWF kankerbestrijding* published a thorough report on cancer in migrants in the year 2006 [10]. It comprises not only the demographics of migrant populations in the Netherlands and projections of future developments but also socio-cultural aspects in the utilization of healthcare services and perception of care.

4.3.5 Possibilities to combine cancer cases and denominator population

In the Netherlands, the proxy for migration background is defined by the same variable in both cancer (numerator, cases) and population data (background population, denominator). Country of birth, as an indicator for migration background, is routinely collected in the NCR and by Statistics Netherlands. Furthermore cancer cases as well as the denominator population are available for the same regions, because of the possibility to exchange data through the electronic network. In addition, important covariables, such as socioeconomic position or treatment, can be taken into account when analysing cancer risks.

In Dutch cancer registry data, the completeness of the country of birth variable varies according to cancer site and is most accurate for deceased patients due to a recheck with municipal population registries. Thus, cancers with low survival and high fatality rates (such as stomach cancer) are assumed to be most complete regarding the country of birth information included in the record. However, cancer mortality data, gathered by the CBS, represent a solid basis for migration-sensitive analyses.

In summary, it is possible to conduct migrant-specific cancer analyses in the Netherlands by means of additional research (surveys, studies), using linkage procedures, but not (yet) within routine analyses.

Citizens service number

Since June 2008, a unique service number (*burgerservicenummer* – BSN) has been assigned to every citizen in the Netherlands and as of 2009 everyone is obligated to use this number in the health sector. It has also been included in the NCR data since mid 2007, without retrospective additions.

This personal identifier has the potential to facilitate linkage procedures of health data (e.g. cancer registry data) and population data, although there is an ongoing debate about the protection of privacy and conforming laws, still inhibiting the utilization of this number in research. It thus remains unclear, when and to what extent this number can in future be used in order to conduct migration-sensitive cancer research. [11]

4.3.6 Conclusion

As an *exemplary* cancer registry (according to our survey), the Netherlands Cancer Registry (NCR) routinely collects country of birth as a proxy for a migration background. It is already relatively easy to conduct migrant-specific analyses as additional research, but not within routine analyses. In the Netherlands, migrant-specific studies on cancer, using cancer registry data have already been successfully done [6, 8-9, 12-13], yielding very interesting and essential findings regarding cancer prevention.

In conclusion, the Netherlands can be seen as an exemplary country because there is a lot of potential for migrant-specific cancer analyses in the future. Population data of good quality on the one, and very good cancer data as well as the potential for exact linkage procedures using the burgerservicenummer on the other hand, are very good prerequisites for migrant-sensitive cancer research. This way, linkage processes between municipalities and cancer registries would be much easier and more resource-efficient.

References
1. CBS_Netherlands, Statline Database. 2010.
2. Rosenau, P.V. and C.J. Lako, An experiment with regulated competition and individual mandates for universal health care: the new Dutch health insurance system. J Health Polit Policy Law, 2008. 33(6): p. 1031-55.
3. IKCnet. KENNISNETWERK integrale kankercentra. 2010; Available from: http://www.ikcnet.nl/.
4. Schouten, L.J., et al., The capture-recapture method for estimation of cancer registry completeness: a useful tool? Int J Epidemiol, 1994. 23(6): p. 1111-6.
5. Schouten, L.J., et al., Completeness of cancer registration in Limburg, The Netherlands. Int J Epidemiol, 1993. 22(3): p. 369-76.
6. Arnold, M., et al., Breast and Stomach Cancer Incidence and Survival in Migrants in the Netherlands, 1989-2006. Eur J Cancer Prev, 2010.
7. Visser, O. and F.E. van Leeuwen, Cancer risk in first generation migrants in North-Holland/Flevoland, The Netherlands, 1995-2004. Eur J Cancer, 2007. 43(5): p. 901-8.
8. Stirbu, I., et al., Cancer mortality rates among first and second generation migrants in the Netherlands: Convergence toward the rates of the native Dutch population. Int J Cancer, 2006. 119(11): p. 2665-72.
9. Bos, V., et al., Ethnic inequalities in age- and cause-specific mortality in The Netherlands. Int J Epidemiol, 2004. 33(5): p. 1112-9.
10. KWF, Allochtonen en Kanker. Socio-culturele en epidemiologische aspecten. 2006, Signaleringscommissie Kanker van KWF Kankerbestrijding
11. Burgerservicenummer (BSN). 2010; Available from: http://www.burgerservicenummer.nl/.
12. Visser, O., et al., Breast cancer risk among first-generation migrants in the Netherlands. Br J Cancer, 2004. 90(11): p. 2135-7.
13. Visser, O., et al., [Incidence of cervical cancer in women in North-Holland by country of birth from 1988-1998]. Ned Tijdschr Geneeskd, 2003. 147(2): p. 70-4.

4.4 Scotland

Melina Arnold[1], David Brewster[2,3]

1   Bielefeld University, Department of Epidemiology and International Public Health, Germany,
2   Scottish Cancer Registry, NHS National Services Scotland, Edinburgh, United Kingdom
3   Edinburgh University Medical School, Edinburgh, United Kingdom

4.4.1 General information about Scotland

Scotland has a total area of 78.772 km². Its population amounts to 5.2 million in 2009. Given the total area, this implies a very low population density of 64 in-habitants per km² (see fig. 4.4.1). Scotland consists of 9 regions and 53 districts, also divisible into 14 National Health Service (NHS) Board areas, 32 council areas and about 1200 communities, including hundreds of islands. [1]

Fig. 4.4.1:   *Population density in Scotland, 2009 [2]*

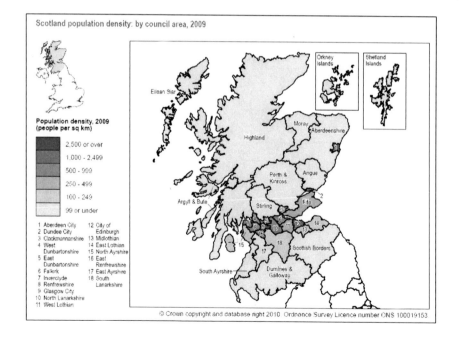

Scotland population density: by council area, 2009

Population density, 2009
(people per sq km)

2,500 or over
1,000 - 2,499
500 - 999
250 - 499
100 - 249
99 or under

1 Aberdeen City
2 Dundee City
3 Clackmannanshire
4 West Dunbartonshire
5 East Dunbartonshire
6 Falkirk
7 Inverclyde
8 Renfrewshire
9 Glasgow City
10 North Lanarkshire
11 West Lothian
12 City of Edinburgh
13 Midlothian
14 East Lothian
15 North Ayrshire
16 East Renfrewshire
17 East Ayrshire
18 South Lanarkshire

© Crown copyright and database right 2010 Ordnance Survey Licence number ONS 100019153

Population

In 2009, Scotland had an estimated mid-year population of 5,194,000, which is the highest since 1981 and still increases slightly from year to year although there is a natural decrease in population (declining fertility and number of births; increasing number of deaths; population aging). This is in large part due to immigration flows coming mainly from the rest of the United Kingdom and EU accession states.

In Scotland, only a small percentage of the population has a migration background that lies outside of Great Britain. 96.2% of Scotland's population was born in the United Kingdom, 87.1% in Scotland, 2.06% in other Western countries (Western Europe, North America, Oceania, Japan) and the remaining 1.70% was born in non-Western countries (referring to the rest of the world). The biggest foreign-born (outside of UK) groups come from Germany (18,703), Pakistan (12,645), the United States (11,149) and India (10,523).

Apart from the Whites, the main foreign ethnic groups originate from South Asia (meaning India, Pakistan, Bangladesh and other) and China. The most recent population census from 2001 recorded 55,007 people of South Asian ethnicity (1.09% of the total population), 16,310 of Chinese ethnicity (0.32% of the total population) and 8,025 people of Black ancestry (0.16% of the total population), see also tab. 4.4.4. [3]

Procedure of the General Register Office for Scotland

The General Register Office for Scotland (GROS) was set up in 1855 and carries responsibility for the registration of events such as births, deaths and marriages. It works closely with the Office for National Statistics in England and Wales. GROS offers extensive data for genealogical purposes dating back to the 15th century.

Conducting a census of the Scottish population every ten years and providing statistics and other demographics for administration, industry as well as research, is the main task of GROS. Census variables include among others ethnicity (1991 and 2001), religion (of upbringing and current) (since 2001), language (since 2001) and country of birth (1991 and 2001). Major ethnic group is categorized into White, Indian, Pakistani and other South Asian, Chinese, Black and other (see tab. 4.4.4). This is especially important with regard to migrant-specific analyses and possible linkage procedures.

Availability of information on ethnicity in Scottish routine health data

In primary care, collecting information on ethnicity is not routine. Historically, there was no common agreement on how to define and code ethnicity in the

General Practice Administration System for Scotland (GPASS), a software that was used in about 85% of all Scottish GP practices. Recording of ethnicity may improve under the auspices of the Primary Care Quality and Outcomes Framework, which rewards general practitioners for recording ethnic origin according to defined categories in newly registering patients.

Tab. 4.4.4: *The size of major and minor ethnic groups according to the Scottish Census 2001 [3]*

Ethnic group according to the Scottish Census 2001					
5 category classification (major ethnic group)	population size	percentage of total population	14 category classification (minor ethnic group)	population size	percentage of total population
White	4.960.334	97,99%	White Scottish	4.459.071	88,09%
			Other White British	373.685	7,38%
			White Irish	49.428	0,98%
			Other White	78.150	1,54%
Indian	15.037	0,30%	Indian	15.037	0,30%
Pakistani and other South Asian	39.970	0,79%	Pakistani	31.793	0,63%
			Bangladeshi	1.981	0,04%
			Other South Asian	6.196	0,12%
Chinese	16.310	0,32%	Chinese	16.310	0,32%
Other	30.360	0,60%	Caribbean	1.778	0,04%
			African	5.118	0,10%
			Black Scottish or other Black	1.129	0,02%
			Any Mixed Background	12.764	0,25%
			Other ethnic group	9.571	0,19%

The Scottish Morbidity Record (SMR-01) scheme records information on hospital episodes and also includes a two character code for ethnic group as an optional, but recommended item. Existing categories should be adapted to the census codes. Information on ethnicity in the SMR-01 is severely incomplete and, for the first quarter of 2009, was missing in 76% of the records. In addition, it is most of the time unclear how data on ethnicity is collected (self-assigned, assigned by staff or relatives?).

Moreover, there are several surveys collecting information on ethnic group like the Scottish Household Survey or the Scottish Longitudinal Study.

In conclusion, Scottish routine health data lacks applicable information regarding ethnicity. If ethnic group is included, it is most often incomplete and not consistent in its categories between studies/databases.

4.4.2 The Scottish healthcare system

NHS Scotland is the main provider of healthcare in Scotland and a separate body from the other public health systems in the United Kingdom. NHS Scotland is solely financed by taxation and free of use for all permanent residents. Primary and secondary healthcare is provided through 14 geographically-based local health boards (NHS boards) and a number of National Special Health Boards which are responsible for the effective and efficient delivery of health services. A wide variety of additional alternative and complementary treatments can be purchased from private healthcare insurances. Patient identification is done via the Community Health Index (CHI), a unique ten-digit number. The Scottish Government's Health and Wellbeing Directorate is in charge of healthcare policy and funding of the system. [4]

4.4.3 Cancer registration in Scotland

The Scottish Cancer Registry

In Scotland, cancer registration has operated since 1958 and was initially carried out by five semi-autonomous regional cancer registries. Their data were compiled in the central Scottish Cancer Registry (SCR) whose function was in the beginning limited to coordination, data collection, analysis and publication. In 1997, this system was reorganized, resulting in one national cancer registry that undertook responsibility for all aspects of registration. The Scottish Cancer Registry is part of the Information Services Division (ISD) of the National Health Service National Services Scotland (NHS NSS) and is staffed by a dedicated team of cancer registration officers located in the main hospitals throughout the country.

The Scottish Cancer Registry collects information on all new cases of primary malignant neoplasms, carcinoma *in situ*, neoplasms of uncertain behaviour and since 2000 benign brain and spinal cord tumours occurring in the population of Scotland. ICD-10 and the second edition of ICD-O were introduced for diagnostic coding of patients diagnosed on and or after January 1997. Previously, records were coded to ICD-9 and morphology to the first edition of ICD-O. The third edition of ICD-O was introduced for patients diagnosed on and or after January 2006. Annual registrations in the registry now exceed 40,000. [5]

Up to the introduction of one single cancer registry in 1997, only a limited data set was collected for each patient. Later, an extended data set became available for all patients including information on the stage of the disease (for breast, colorectal and cervical cancer), treatment details, method of first detection, grade of differentiation and entry to any clinical trial. Although ethnicity was also added as a new variable to the data sets, its completeness is still insufficient and only poorly recorded (over 80% of cases with "unknown ethnicity").

In order to monitor the data quality, routine indicators, computer validation and ad hoc studies of data accuracy and completeness of ascertainment are applied. The Scottish Open Cancer Registration and Tumour Enumeration System (SOCRATES) is a computer system receiving notification of cancer from hospital systems, including discharges (SMR01 records), radiotherapy, oncology, haematology and pathology records, prospective audit datasets, deaths from the General Register Office of Scotland and paper records from private hospitals. This information is linked to create provisional registrations that are passed on to the competent cancer registration officers. Validating these provisional records as well as adding additional information is the main task of these staff. During this active process, data quality can be assured and sustained.

A new, web based version of SOCRATES which includes some important new features like enhanced validation was launched in June 2006. Presently, methods to improve data linkage procedures are being developed in order to extend the range of source data and thereby introduce new analysis options and possibilities for research.

Ascertainment of cases by the Scottish Cancer Registry is believed to be reasonably complete. Routine indicators of data quality, such as the percentage of registrations based on a death certificate only (DCO) support this conclusion. For example, during the period of diagnosis 1998-2002, the DCO percentage for all cancers excluding non-melanoma skin cancer was less than 1% [6]. Ad hoc studies also suggest that ascertainment is relatively complete for most cancer sites [7-9].

Population based cancer registration

The Scottish Cancer Registry covers the whole country with its about five million inhabitants. Most cancer patients are diagnosed and receive their primary therapy at district general hospitals. Cancer registrations are electronically identified through hospital discharge, oncology, pathology and death records.

Available data in the cancer registry

The Scottish Cancer Registry routinely collects data on demographic information of a patient. Age at diagnosis is derived from date of birth and date of incidence. A real indicator for socioeconomic status is constructed by use of the area of residence and census variables. Ethnicity is based on the Scottish Census categories and only complete in about 18% of the cancer patients due to missing information in medical records.

Furthermore, hospital data, data on the diagnosis of the tumour as well as treatment and follow-up information are registered.

- Demographic data:
  - first name and surname (as well as change of name)
  - sex
  - date of birth (date, month, year)
  - place of residence (address, postal code)
  - ethnic group according to predefined categories from the Scottish Census
  - unique person identifier
- Hospital data:
  - hospital of diagnosis
- Data on diagnosis of tumour:
  - source of information
  - tumour site and type
  - date of incidence, date of diagnosis
  - basis and certainty of the diagnosis
  - method of first detection
  - topography and laterality, the localisation of the tumour
  - morphology, tissue typing
  - TNM for some cancers
  - tumour histology
- Treatment data:
  - type of treatment (surgery, radiotherapy, chemotherapy, hormone therapy, other therapy)
  - hospital of treatment
- Follow-up data:
  - cause of death
  - date of death
  - date of emigration
  - entry to any clinical trial

4.4.4 Migrant-specific cancer research

In Scotland, information on ethnicity in routine health data is rather poor. Existing data is incomplete and its coding most of the time not consistent between data sources. Preferably, data on ethnicity should be collected according to the Scottish census classification and first attempts have been made to achieve this. Since data acquisition concerning ethnicity is challenging and not satisfactory coupled with the fact that ethnic minorities are (still) relatively small in Scotland (compared to other parts of the United Kingdom, for example), only very little research has been conducted on ethnicity and cancer in Scotland till now. The "retrocoding project", based on linkage of ethnic codes from the census to the

SMR-01 database, is a novel approach that will allow migrant specific cancer research in the future.

Epidemiology of cancer in ethnic groups [10]

Muir reviews studies on cancer in migrant groups that have been conducted in the United Kingdom and the United States. He refers to a study of Harkness (1993; retrieved via personal communication) that examined nasopharyngeal cancer occurring in the Chinese of Scotland. 213 cases of this tumour could be identified in the Scottish Cancer Registry and using a name-based approach, 7.5% of those were found out to be Chinese, while the proportion of Chinese in the Scottish population was 0.2% at that time. Calculating age-standardised incidence rates resulted in 0.3 per 100,000 population for the entire Scottish population and 13.7 for persons with Chinese names (RR=46). This figure is close to that of Chinese minorities elsewhere.

Cancer in Italian migrant populations. Scotland [11]

Black observed significantly increased rates of stomach cancer among males born in Italy compared to the Scottish population. Moreover, he found a lower mortality of lung cancer in Italy-born males and females, whereas laryngeal cancer was significantly commoner in Italian males compared to Scottish males. Mortality from cancers of the breast, uterus and ovary were consistently lower in Italian females, although this association was not statistically significant.

Oral carcinoma in the Indian and Pakistani community in Scotland [12]

Merchant et al. investigated the occurrence of oral carcinoma and its relation to betel and tobacco consumption in the South Asian population of Scotland. Data on cancer incidence was obtained from the Scottish Cancer Registry for the period 1968-1978 and people of Indian/ Pakistani origin were identified based on their first names and surnames. 64 cases of malignant tumours were recorded in this migrant group, two of oral carcinoma. Age-adjusted relative frequencies for oral cancer, lung cancer in males and breast cancer in females were calculated and compared to registry data of Bombay and the total Scottish population. The relative frequency for oral carcinoma was considerably lower in the Scottish Indian/Pakistani population compared to the rate from Bombay and was close to that of the total Scottish population. The relative frequencies for lung cancer in males and breast cancer in females in Scottish South Asians were midway between the frequencies found in Bombay and Scotland overall. In addition, a high frequency of lymphoma (13.4%) was observed in Scottish South Asians, relative to both Bombay and total Scottish figures.

Incidence of colorectal, breast and lung cancer in a Scottish Asian population [13]

In their study on cancer in the Asian population in the West of Scotland aged 45-64 years, Matheson et al. found significantly lower incidences of colorectal, breast and lung cancer compared to the indigenous population. The authors ascribe this difference in risk to dietary factors and refer mainly to lacto-vegetarian diets and meat consumption, prevailing in the Scottish Asian minority. During their study period from 1961 to 1981, they also observed an increased risk for cervical cancer in Scottish Asian women which is consistent with previous findings implying that women from underdeveloped countries tend to have a higher incidence of cervical cancer compared to women from Western countries. The comparison of the cancer incidence rates of Scottish Asians obtained during the study period to incidence data from Bombay, India, revealed a greater degree of coherence. This means that the rates of the Scottish Asian population are closer to those of their home than to those of their host country.

Scottish Asians were previously identified based on their names and medical records were used to confirm the ethnic origin of each patient. An additional cross check was conducted by collecting death certificates from the Registrar General to estimate the accuracy of the name-based approach.

4.4.5 Possibilities to combine cancer cases and denominator population

In Scotland, ethnicity is only recorded accurately in the Scottish population census where it is defined as described in chapter 3.2. Medical records are intended to include the same categories as used in the census but are very incomplete and not reliable.

Mortality data do not include ethnicity, but do include country of birth, which has been used to study patterns of cancer in migrants in England and Wales [14-15] and patterns of all cause and cardiovascular mortality in Scotland [16].

Again, since data on cancer in migrant populations is very incomplete in Scotland, analyses are not feasible directly in the Scottish Cancer Registry. However, there are possibilities to conduct migrant-specific research by use of linkage procedures which has already been tested in a pilot project by Fischbacher and colleagues and has recently been further explored by Bhopal and colleagues [17].

Linkage studies

For the first time, Fischbacher et al. [17-18] linked information on ethnicity from the 2001 Scottish Population Census to Scottish hospital discharge and mortality data (SMR01). This was done by means of the Community Health Index (CHI), a unique person identifier that is also included in health records. The linkage was performed using probability matching (taking into account date of birth, surname, forename, address and full postcode) and encryption methods in such a way as to preserve confidentiality. In the end, for 94% of the records, an ethnicity code could be ascribed which is slightly less than normally achieved within ISD (around 98%).

The authors used CHD as outcome, but the very same steps can also in future be applied for cancers [16, 18-19].

Only recently, Bhopal and colleagues [17] confirmed the feasibility of linkage studies with Scottish health data in a second phase, extracting information on ethnicity as well as other relevant variables from the 2001 census, and demonstrating the application in different settings and with different outcomes. In this way, not only cancer occurrence but also use of prevention measures and care services use can be evaluated, following this method.

Currently, there are no studies carried out in the Scottish Cancer Registry that deal with migrant populations. There are though plans to conduct analyses on ethnic minorities such as investigating differences in cancer risk, breast screening uptake, stage distribution, use of treatment and survival in the future.

Based on the findings of the above named studies, migrant-specific cancer analyses using linkage procedures are possible and highly expedient in Scotland.

The Community Health Index (CHI) number

In Scotland, the so called Community Health Index (CHI) number, a population register, is used for health care purposes and uniquely identifies every person that is registered with a Scottish GP and making use of the Scottish health care system. More than 99% of the Scottish population is listed. It is presently being added to the Master Patient Indexes and preserving privacy whilst making names less important is one of the major goals. The current CHI number consists of the six digit date of birth (DDMMYY) followed by a three digit sequence number and a check digit. The ninth digit is always even for females and odd for males. The CHI number is associated with important health-related factors (like immunization status, screening participation and risk behaviour, but also prescription exemptions and prepayment codes) as well as other demographics of the patient (such as name, address, date of birth, postcode, etc). [20]

The CHI can be used as the Hospital Patient Identifier (Case Reference Number) and is mainly used for record linkage purposes, for example to the SMR02 (maternity inpatient and day case), and the SMR11 (neonatal inpatient) or SMR01 (general/acute inpatient and day case), and also for linkage between SMR00 (outpatient attendance) and SMR01. In the long run it may be an important step in reducing the number of patient identifying items routinely included on SMR returns.

The CHI is an excellent instrument to facilitate epidemiologic research and bears many advantages with regard to migrant-specific analyses. Since ethnicity as well as country of birth is included in the Scottish census, linkage to morbidity and mortality data based on the CHI has approved to be a good option and overturned the expectations after completion of the pilot phase which focused on CHD but is in the same manner feasible for cancer or other major diseases. [21]

4.4.6 Conclusion

So far, there has only been very limited research on cancer in migrants in Scotland. This may be due to relatively small numbers of migrants represented in the Scottish population. In fact, ethnic diversity is expected to increase gradually and recent immigrants tend to be from more diverse backgrounds than immigrants in the past. Growing ethnic minorities have different health care needs and may challenge existing systems. The availability of reliable data is one of the most important prerequisites for addressing and meeting those needs. [22]

Existing Scottish studies on cancer risk of migrants revealed significant differences between ethnic minorities and the native Scottish population and underline the importance of migrant-specific research.

In fact, there has been progress in terms of data linkage and consequently facilitation of migrant-specific research on a more routine basis. Presently, convergence of definitions and categories of ethnicity in Scottish health data is taking place, following the comprehensive definition of the Scottish Census. Still, most health records lack completeness of this variable which makes research almost impossible.

The CHI has been proven to be a good instrument to conduct migrant-specific research. Its utility and the possibility to link data from the census to routine health databases in a way that preserves privacy has been tested successfully using data on cardiovascular diseases in South Asian migrants. Fischbacher et al. [18] thereby confirmed that migrant-specific analyses are feasible at relatively low costs and within a reasonable time frame. This "breakthrough" should provide future incentives for research and appeal to researchers in this field. In the long run, a similar linkage approach for data on cancer in migrant groups can be performed. Results imply a high relevance to policy makers, future research, planners, clinical networks, service providers.

References
1. Wikipedia. Scotland. 2010; Available from: http://en.wikipedia.org/wiki/Scotland.
2. ONS, UK National Statistics. 2010, Office of National Statistics UK.

3.   GROS. General Register Office for Scotland. 2010; Available from: http://www.gro-scotland.gov.uk/.
4.   NHS_Scotland. About the NHS in Scotland. 2010; Available from: http://www.show.scot.nhs.uk/introduction.aspx.
5.   ISD. Information Services Devision Scotland – Cancer Information Programme. 2010; Available from: http://www.isdscotland.org/isd/338.html.
6.   IARC, Cancer incidence in five continents. Volume IX. IARC Sci Publ, 2008(160): p. 1-837.
7.   Brewster, D.H., et al., Completeness of case ascertainment in a Scottish regional cancer registry for the year 1992. Public Health, 1997. 111(5): p. 339-43.
8.   Brewster, D.H. and D.L. Stockton, Ascertainment of breast cancer by the Scottish Cancer Registry: an assessment based on comparison with five independent breast cancer trials databases. Breast, 2008. 17(1): p. 104-6.
9.   Melia, J., et al., Problems with registration of cutaneous malignant melanoma in England. Br J Cancer, 1995. 72(1): p. 224-8.
10. Muir, C.S., Epidemiology of cancer in ethnic groups. Br J Cancer Suppl, 1996. 29: p. S12-6.
11. Black, R.J., Cancer in Italian migrant populations. Scotland. IARC Sci Publ, 1993(123): p. 186-92.
12. Merchant, N.E., et al., Oral carcinoma in the Indian and Pakistani community in Scotland. J Oral Med, 1986. 41(1): p. 62-5.
13. Matheson, L.M., et al., Incidence of colo-rectal, breast and lung cancer in a Scottish Asian population. Health Bull (Edinb), 1985. 43(5): p. 245-9.
14. Wild, S.H., et al., Mortality from all cancers and lung, colorectal, breast and prostate cancer by country of birth in England and Wales, 2001-2003. Br J Cancer, 2006. 94(7): p. 1079-85.
15. Harding, S., M. Rosato, and A. Teyhan, Trends in cancer mortality among migrants in England and Wales, 1979-2003. Eur J Cancer, 2009. 45(12): p. 2168-79.
16. Fischbacher, C., et al., Variations in all cause and cardiovascular mortality by country of birth in Scotland, 1997-2003. Scottish Medical Journal, 2007. 52(4): p. 5-10.
17. Bhopal, R., et al., Cohort profile: Scottish Health and Ethnicity Linkage Study of 4.65 million people exploring ethnic variations in disease in Scotland. Int J Epidemiol, 2010.
18. Fischbacher, C.M., et al., Record linked retrospective cohort study of 4.6 million people exploring ethnic variations in disease: myocardial infarction in South Asians. BMC Public Health, 2007. 7: p. 142.
19. Bhopal, R., et al. (2005) Ethnicity and health in Scotland: can we fill the information gap? A demonstration project focusing on coronary heart disease and linkage of census and health records.
20. Womersley, J., The public health uses of the Scottish Community Health Index (CHI). Journal of public health medicine, 1996. 18(4): p. 465-472.
21. NHS. CHI / Community Health Index 2006; Available from: http://www.nhsgg.org.uk/content/default.asp?page=home_chi.
22. Bhopal, R.S., Ethnicity, Race, and Health in Multicultural Societies: Foundations for Better Epidemiology, Public Health, and Health Care. 2007: Oxford Univ Pr.

4.5 Sweden

Omid Beiki[1,2,3], Birgitta Stegmayr[4], Tahereh Moradi[5]

1   Karolinska Institutet, Clinical Epidemiology Unit, Department of Medicine, Stockholm, Sweden.
2   Kermanshah University of Medical Sciences, Kermanshah, Iran.
3   Yazd Shahid Sadoughi University of Medical Sciences, Yazd, Iran.
4   The National Board of Health and Welfare, Stockholm, Sweden.
5   Karolinska Institutet, Institute of Environmental Medicine, Division of Epidemiology, Stockholm, Sweden.

Sweden was included in the survey as exemplary country since there are unique possibilities for conducting nation-wide epidemiological studies among immigrants. First, country of birth for the entire population of Sweden is registered in population registers on behalf of the Swedish Tax Agency [1]. Second, Sweden has a number of high-quality national registers in different areas including health and demographic registers, collected via different agencies. And finally, these register could be linked using the unique personal identification number that introduced in 1947 for everybody residing longer than one year in Sweden [2].

4.5.1 General information about Sweden

Sweden is one of the largest countries in the European Union in terms of area with 450 thousands square kilometres and a population around 9 million corresponding to a low population density of 21 inhabitants per square kilometre. Compared with the other parts of the country, the southern part of Sweden has a considerably higher population density. The majority of the Swedish population lives in urban areas. Sweden is divided into 21 counties including 290 municipalities and 2,512 parishes (fig. 4.5.1).

Population

By the end of 2008, Sweden's population was estimated to be 9,256,347. During the year 2008, the population had increased by 73,000 persons, corresponding to the highest increase during one year since 1970. Immigration accounted for 76 percent and new births for 24 percent of the population increase.

Net migration to Sweden has been positive since the 1930s. This is mainly due to a substantial increase of foreign-born people coming to and residing in Sweden. In 1900, less than one per cent of the Swedish population was born in a foreign country, whereas in 2008, 13.8% was born abroad. This group of immigrants currently comprises 200 different nationalities. The majority (56.9%) of foreign-born population are European with 21.0% coming from other Scandinavian countries. Asia, Africa, South America, and North America accounts for 28.2%, 7.1%, 4.8%, and 2.2% of the foreign-born population, respectively.

The countries representing the largest immigrant groups are Finland with 13.7%, Iraq with 8.5%, former Federal Republic of Yugoslavia with 5.6%, Poland with 5.0%, and Iran with 4.5% of the foreign-born population in Sweden (tab. 4.5.1) [5]. According to the population projection by Statistics Sweden, the proportion of foreign-born persons is expected to rise to around 18.5 percent in 2050 (fig. 4.5.2, p. 109). In 2008, Sweden-born individuals with two foreign-born parents accounted for 4.1% of total population in Sweden.

Fig. 4.5.1: *(a) Counties and municipalities, (b) Population density by municipality of Sweden. Sources: Statistics Sweden/SCB and Wikipedia [3-4]*

a   b

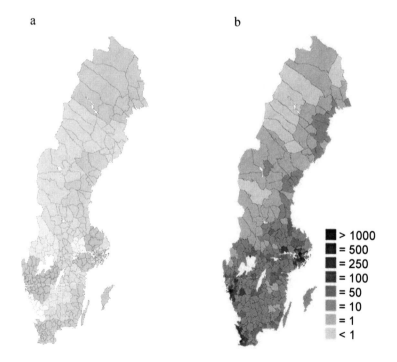

> 1000
= 500
= 250
= 100
= 50
= 10
= 1
< 1

Population registration in Sweden

People who are born in Sweden or who move to Sweden and live there for at least one year should normally be registered in The Swedish Population Register to provide reliable information for various purposes such as programme planning, budgeting and taxation; for population estimation, census planning, and census evaluation and for sampling frame of household surveys. Hence, people that leave Sweden and are away for at least one year should normally be excluded from the population register. Every person registered in Sweden is allocated a 10 digits unique Personal Identification Number (PIN). The first six digits indicate the date of birth (year, month, day) and the last four are check digits (fig. 4.5.3). A person who has once been given a PIN will retain that number for life. In other words, the PIN will not be altered, for example in case of emigration or re-immigration.

Tab. 4.5.1: *Immigrants registered in Sweden between 1960 and 2007 [4]*

Birth Region	No. Population	Birth Region	No. Population
Africa	110,162	Ex-Soviet Union	36,842
Northern Africa	22,637	other	6,972
Western Africa	17,205	Northern Europe	677,037
Other Africa	70,320	Denmark	103,222
Ethiopia	14,851	Estonia	26,006
Somalia	29,942	Finland	372,160
other	25,527	Iceland	13,491
Asia	463,162	Norway	111,704
Eastern Asia	46,902	UK	35,266
China	24,680	other	15,188
Korea (Republic)	11,845	Southern Europe	238,492
other	10,377	Bosnia	62,050
South-Central Asia	127,935	Greece	25,503
Afghanistan	11,977	Italy	16,036
India	19,935	Spain	12,453
Iran	68,974	Ex-Yugoslavia	116,358
other	27,049	other	6,092
South-Eastern Asia	60,702	Western Europe	135,832
Thailand	28,013	Austria	11,889
Viet Nam	14,934	France	14,859
other	17,755	Germany	86,530
Western Asia	227,623	Netherlands	12,988
Iraq	114,933	other	9,566
Lebanon	26,542	Latin America	89,378
Syria	20,215	South America	76,406
Turkey	46,703	Colombia	11,083
other	19,230	Chile	34,731
Europe	1,232,752	other	30,592
Eastern Europe	181,391	Central/Caribbean	12,972
Ex-Czechoslovakia	14,280	Northern America	47,412
Hungary	23,297	Canada	5,742
Poland	79,228	USA	41,601
Romania	20,772	Oceania	8,631

With the introduction of national registers, the PIN has become a vital component of for research purposes [2] where the PIN is used as the linkage tool between various health and demographic data.

Fig. 4.5.2:   *Current projection of population change in Sweden [4]*

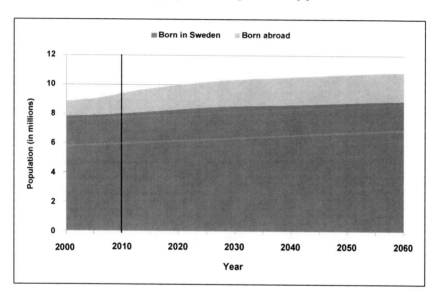

Fig. 4.5.3:   *Personal Identity Number in Sweden [1]*

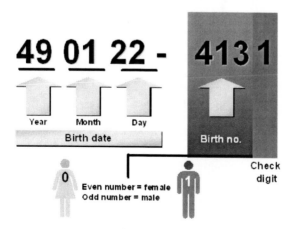

The Swedish Tax Agency is responsible for population registration in Sweden that is registered in The Population Register and includes information on:

- Name
- Personal identity number and co-ordination number
- Place of birth, in Sweden or abroad
- Citizenship
- Civil status
- Spouse, children, parents, guardian(s) and adoption
- Address
- Property, parish and municipality
- Date of Immigration to and emigration from Sweden
- Address abroad
- Death and place of burial.

Statistics Sweden was established in 1858. The tasks of Statistics Sweden are to develop, produce and disseminate statistics and coordinate and support the Swedish system for official statistics. Statistics Sweden is also responsible for producing official statistics in a number of different areas including labour market, population, housing, living conditions, environment, education and research.

In the area of population statistics, SCB gives an annual picture of population size and changes in the population, with regard to births, deaths, domestic and foreign migration. These statistics are based on the Swedish Population Register, which extracts data from the tax agency's population registration list. Statistics Sweden also provides details of the composition of the population by sex, age, civil status, country of birth and citizenship for entire Sweden as well as its counties, municipalities and urban areas. The former population and housing censuses (1960-1990) are included in this statistical area [6-7].

Tab. 4.5.2: *The Statistics Sweden definition of foreign and Swedish background [8]*

Persons with foreign background	Persons with Swedish background
Born outside Sweden with two parents born outside Sweden	Born outside-Sweden with at least one parent born in Sweden
Born in-Sweden with two parents born outside Sweden	Born in-Sweden with one parent born in Sweden and one parent born outside Sweden
	Born in-Sweden with two parents born in Sweden

Availability of information on country of birth, ethnicity and foreign background Country of birth of an immigrant can be extracted from The Swedish Population Register mentioned above. Concerning the term "foreign background", Statistics Sweden has published directions how to code national origin in scientific studies, based on a person's immigration status and citizenship (tab.

4.5.2). However, researchers might select different ways of defining a foreign background. At present, there is no possibility to retrieve any information on ethnicity from official statistics in Sweden.

4.5.2 The Swedish healthcare system

Sweden has a decentralized health care system which is mainly funded by taxes, with nominal fees for patients. Twenty-one county councils, embedded in six health care regions (fig. 4.5.4), are responsible for supplying their citizens with health care services. They are regulated by the Health and Medical Service Act (Hälso- och sjukvårdslagen, HSL). The central government established principles and guidelines for care and sets the political agenda for health and medical care. A person seeking care first contacts a clinic for a doctor's appointment, and may then be referred to a specialist by the clinic physician, who may in turn recommend either in-patient or out-patient treatment, or an elective care option.

Fig. 4.5.4:   Six medical regions of Sweden

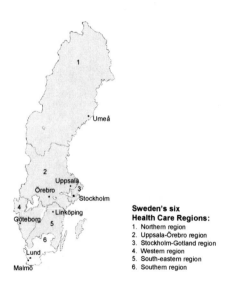

Sweden's six
Health Care Regions:
1. Northern region
2. Uppsala-Örebro region
3. Stockholm-Gotland region
4. Western region
5. South-eastern region
6. Southern region

Source: National Board of Health and Welfare, Sweden.

Since 2005, there is a health care guarantee in Sweden, meaning that no patient has to wait more than 90 days for being treated once a diagnosis and treatment plan has been determined.

4.5.3 Cancer registration in Sweden

The Swedish Cancer Register

The Swedish Cancer Register was founded in 1958 and covers all persons diagnosed with cancer in Sweden. This allows the extensive description of cancer patterns as well as analyses of cancer trends and survival. Approximately 50,000 malignant cases of cancer are being registered in Sweden every year. It is compulsory for every health care provider to report newly detected cancer cases diagnosed during clinical, pathological, morphological or other laboratory examinations as well as cases diagnosed at autopsy to the cancer registry.

New cancer reports are registered through six regional cancer registries in the country (fig. 4.5.4). These registries are associated with the oncological centers in each medical region of Sweden, where the registration, coding, major checkup and corrections are being performed in close contact with the reporting physician. The regional registers send information of newly registered cases and corrections of previously reported cases to the Swedish Cancer Register at the National Board of Health and Welfare on an annual basis.

The following diseases are to be reported to the Swedish Cancer Register:
A. All definitely malignant neoplasms (e.g. carcinoma, sarcoma, malignant lymphoma, leukemia and malignant teratoma).
B. Carcinoid tumors of digestive and other organs, granulose cell tumors of the ovary, thymomas, adamantinomas and chordomas.
C. Histologically benign tumors of the central nervous system and meninges, transitional cell papillomas of the urinary tract, all hormonally active tumors of the endocrine glands (except the thyroid) and the entero-chromaffin and neuroendocrine systems.
D. Precancerous lesions of lip, mouth, larynx, bronchus, trachea, cervix uteri, skin, vulva and vagina, gastro-intestinal polyps with suspected malignancy, "bronchial adenomas", atypical epithelial proliferations of the breast (carcinoma in situ type) and adenoma phyllodes, precancerous endometrial lesions, hydatidiform moles of placental tissue, and ovarian cystadenomas of borderline type.

If a person has more than one primary tumor, each tumor is registered separately.

Data available in the Swedish Cancer Register

There are three different types of information registered in the cancer register:
• Data on the patient
  – Personal identification number

- Sex
- Age
- Place of residence.
• Medical data
  - Site of tumour: For the years 1987-1992 the tumours have primarily been coded in ICD-9 and from 1993-2004 in ICD-O/2. From 2005 the cases has been coded in ICD-O/3. For the whole period from 1958 the codes are available as ICD-7 codes.
  - Histological type
  - Stage: available from 2004
  - Basis of diagnosis: only clinical examination, radiology or histology/cytology confirmed
  - Date of diagnosis
  - Reporting hospital and department
  - Reporting pathology/cytology department
  - Identification number for the tissue specimen.
• Follow-up data
  - Date of death
  - Cause of death
  - Date of migration.

Quality of the Swedish Cancer Register

To preserve the data quality, the collected information is checked in different steps. The first step is checking the PIN against the Swedish Population Register of Sweden. Further steps imply a special check for duplicates, validity and logical contents of the codes. A couple of studies aiming to evaluate the quality of the cancer register have been conducted [9-12]. The overall completeness of cases in the Cancer registry was high for most cancers but was lower for some type of cancers such as renal pelvic and urethral carcinomas, and indolent lympho-proliferative tumours. A recent article evaluating the coverage rate against the inpatient register, estimated the underreporting to be around 4 percent [9]. It was concluded that the overall completeness of the register is high and underreporting will not have any major impact for most uses in epidemiological studies.

Since the Swedish Cancer Register does not include notifications from death certificates, an estimation of the underreporting of cancers was also performed by comparing the Cancer Register data with the Cause of Death Register. It was concluded that underreporting was highly dependent on the cancer site; for example breast cancer has very low underreporting while a larger number of pancreatic and lung cancers are not reported to the cancer register due to a low rate of biopsy performed in these sites [9]. The decreasing autopsy rates in Sweden may also result in underestimation of cancer cases not being discovered.

The National Health Care Quality Registries

A system of national quality registries has been established in the Swedish health and medical services in the last decade. The Swedish Association of Local Authorities and Regions (SALAR) and the National Board of Health and Welfare have collaborated for more than a decade to support the development and use of National Quality Registries. Since 2007, the local authorities and regions such as county councils have taken on the primary responsibility for the continuing operation, development, and financing of the registries. The registries are being developed and managed by professional representatives. From around 15 registries in the early 1990s, Sweden has now more than 60 registers that receive financial support via the Executive Committee.

These registries contain individual based data on diagnoses, treatments and outcomes. The following National Quality Registers relate to cancer [13]:

National Prostate Cancer Registry

The National Prostate Cancer Registry covers 97.5% of all prostate cancer cases compared to the National Cancer Registry and incorporates data from all departments that diagnose and treat prostate cancer. In 2005, the registry reported 9,548 new cases of prostate cancer.

National Breast Cancer Registry

Register began to be used regionally in Stockholm-Gotland region in 2007 and nationally in 2008. All new cases of primary invasive and non invasive breast cancer in women and men are registered. Coverage after one year of registration was high, and over 7,000 cases registered.

National Quality Registry for Oesophageal and Stomach Cancer

In 2007, 55 surgery and oncology departments participated in the registry under written agreements between the unit directors and the registry. When checked against the cancer registry, data processed manually indicate that just over 50% are registered.

Swedish Rectal Cancer Registry

Every patient with rectal cancer is registered. All units participate, and coverage exceeds 99%. Registration is verified with the oncology centres in each region, where reporting is linked to the cancer registry. Hence, all rectal cancers are captured. Annually, around 1500 patients contract the disease.

Swedish Gyn-Oncology Registry

All gynaecology units in Sweden, oncology centres, and the Swedish Society of Obstetrics & Gynaecology are represented in the working group for the registry. Issues concerning the level of coverage and missing patients can be addressed by checking against the cancer registry. However, no report on the coverage is currently available. Each year, around 3,000 cases of gynaecological cancer are reported to the cancer registry.

Swedish Colon Cancer Registry

All patients with adenocarcinoma in the colon are registered. This will be possible since all hospitals that offer colon cancer surgery have agreed to participate. The National Registry of colon cancer, started 1 January 2007 and no information about its coverage has been reported yet.

4.5.4 Migration-sensitive cancer research

There are a number of migrant studies on cancer risk and mortality utilizing data from the Swedish Cancer Register. Most of these studies are based on data from two different databases established through linkages between different Swedish registers.

The first database, Health and Migration Cohort, designed specifically to address the health status of immigrants and their descendants as well as of social disadvantaged groups in Sweden. This database was created by linkages between fifteen Swedish national demographic and health registers in order to study cancer, injuries, diabetes, cardiovascular and psychiatric diseases in these groups. The Health and Migration Cohort covers the total population of Sweden and includes data from the following nation-wide registers:

1. The Swedish Population Register with information such as country of birth, immigration and emigration dates and current residence including county and municipality;
2. The National Population and Housing Censuses 1960-1990 cover demographic, occupational and socioeconomic factors such as income, occupation and education for each household member;
3. The Longitudinal Integration Database for Health Insurance and Labour Market studies (LISA) since 1990 includes several demographic, occupational, and socioeconomic factors such as individual income, family income, capital income, education, and marital status. LISA contains for every year specification on: income from different sources, attained level of education, place of living and working;

4. Multi-generation Register which contains information of all individuals about family relationships, country of birth and reproductive history since 1932.
5. The Cause of Death Register contains information on date of death and underlying cause of death since 1952;
6. The In-patient Register, from 1987, includes all in-patient care in Sweden and includes 50 million discharges for the period 1964 to 2006.
7. The Outpatient Register contains, from 2001, outpatient visits including day surgery and psychiatric from both private and public caregivers. Primary care is not yet covered;
8. The Cancer Register containing data on all cases of cancer since 1958;
9. Register on prescribed pharmaceuticals contains individual data for all drugs prescribed and dispensed to whole population of Sweden since 2005;
10. The Swedish Medical Birth Register was started in 1973 in order to collect data on antenatal and perinatal factors and their importance for the health of the infant, variables and contains information such as maternal age, caesarean section delivery, gestational age, and birth weight.
11. The National Myocardial Infarction Register containing all 336 000 cases of first MI that occurred since 1995;
12. The Swedish Coronary Angiography and Angioplasty register (SCAAR) created in 1991 which register PCI procedures performed in Sweden;
13. The Register of information and knowledge about Swedish Intensive Heart Care admissions (RIKS-HIA) started nationally 1995 with 21 participating hospitals. RIKS-HIA registers all patients admitted to the coronary care units of all participating hospitals;
14. The Swedish Heart Surgery Register contains information on open heart surgeries since 1992.
15. The Stockholm breast cancer quality register.

The information in the Health and Migration Cohort is updated continuously to cover the changes of population such as birth, death, immigration and emigration as well as new diagnosis. Examples of studies that used this database are by Beiki and Moradi [14-17].

The second database, the Family-Cancer Database, is created by linking the Swedish multi-generation cancer register with national census of 1960, 1970, 1980 and 1990 [18]. Main purpose of this database was to study familial cancer risk in Sweden. For this reason the database includes only individuals who are a parent of a child born in Sweden. Later, researchers used this database to perform migrant studies. Since the probability of having a child is not the same among native Swedes and immigrants [19] and because it has been shown that the risk of some cancers is influenced by reproductive factors, this kind of selection might be a source of bias in migrant studies using data from this register. Studies performed by Hemminki and Mousavi are from this database [18, 20-23].

Cancer Incidence rates among immigrants

Comparison with rates in the host country

Almost all migrant studies that have been conducted until now include the comparison of incidence rates among immigrants to that among native Swedes.

Only few studies were performed without focusing on a specific migrant group or a specific cancer type [18, 20, 22]. However, the comparison of cancer rates between foreign-born and native Swedes resulted in lower all-cancer incidence rates of 8% and 5% for immigrant women and men, respectively. Conversely, a 41% increase in lung cancer among male migrants was observed. Among individual cancer sites and immigrant countries, 110 comparisons were statistically significant, 62 showing a protective and 48 an increased risk [20].

Comparison with rates in the country of origin

Nilsson and colleagues [24] studied the cancer incidence among Estonian immigrants in Sweden as compared to the cancer risk of the total Swedish population and that of Estonians in Estonia using the Swedish and the Estonian cancer registries. Male lung cancer and stomach cancer showed a higher incidence in the Estonian population than in the Swedish- and in the migrant populations. The migrant population had an intermediate incidence relative to Estonians in Estonia and to the entire Swedish population. This implies the importance of environmental factors in the aetiology of cancers. However, in contrast with the findings of other studies of an intermediate risks between the country of origin and the host country among immigrants, the risk of the cancer of colon in Estonian migrants in Sweden was higher than the risk in Estonians in Estonia and the risk in the Swedish population.

In a study conducted at the Karolinska Institutet, Beiki and colleagues compared prostate cancer incidence rates among foreign-born and Swedish-born men in Sweden and among men residing in the countries of origin in nine selected countries using the Health & Migration Cohort [15]. The rate of prostate cancer among all immigrants as one group, as well as the rates among immigrants for the selected countries was lower compared to Swedish-born men. Except for immigrants from Estonia and the USA, the country-specific trends were similar to that of the trend among immigrants as one group. Furthermore, immigrants from Denmark, Germany and UK had a pattern similar to that of residents of their countries of origin. Immigrants from Estonia and USA had a more similar pattern to Swedish-born men [15]. These observations indicate the importance of both genetic factors and modifiable environmental factors in the etiology of prostate cancer.

Recently, two studies were conducted to compare cancer risks among Iranian immigrants to the native Swedish population and to Iranian residents. Mousavi and colleagues used The Swedish Family-Cancer Database to get information on Iranian immigrants and native Swedes [23]. They also extracted data for Iranian residents from the Iranian cancer registry which registers only pathological records using a cross-sectional method. Higher all-cancer incidence rates were found among Iranian immigrants compared to Iranian residents. By contrast, the all-cancers risk in Iranian immigrants was found to be lower than that in the native Swedish population. In the second study, Zendehdel and colleagues [25] followed a cohort of Iranian immigrants in Sweden from 1960 to 2004 through record linkages with Swedish registers of cancer, death, and migration. They compared age-standardized incidence rates and estimated Standard Rate Ratios for various cancer sites among Iranian immigrants with corresponding rates from Iran (Tehran capital city) and Sweden. The Tehran Cancer Registry (TCR) was used for cancer rates in Iran. A validation study of the TCR reported 25% underreporting (unpublished report). A significantly different incidence rates for stomach, breast, and non-melanoma skin cancer were observed among female Iranian immigrants in as well as for oesophageal, stomach, colorectal, and prostate cancers among male Iranian immigrants in Sweden in comparison to the rates reported in the Tehran Cancer Registry.

Moradi and colleagues conducted a registry-based study of Swedish residents born in Iran on thyroid cancer [17]. The relative risks of thyroid cancer adjusted for attained age, calendar year of period and education among Iranian immigrants were 2.6 compared to native Swedes. In both sexes, the excess risk was highest among people who were younger than 30 years at immigration. The incidence rate ratio was higher among subjects who immigrated before 1990 than among those immigrated thereafter, particularly among men. Iodine deficiency, increased surveillance of especially young women, and exposure to environmental risk factors including ionizing radiation early in life are possible explanations for these findings.

Studies on the effect of age at immigration or duration of residence

A couple of studies on the effect of age at immigration and duration of residence have already been conducted in Sweden. Beiki and colleagues investigated the risk of gynaecologic cancers among foreign-born women compared to Swedish-born women in a cohort of 5.3 million women between 1969 and 2004 [14]. They found that the adjusted relative risks of all three gynaecologic cancers were lower or equal among foreign-born women compared to women born in

Sweden. Overall, the risk of cervical cancer increased with higher age at migration but there was no variation in relative risks for cervical cancer by duration of residence in all immigrant groups combined (fig. 4.5.5). In another study by Azerkan and colleagues the risk of invasive cervical cancer among immigrant women was studied. Follow-up time as well as age at migration were found to be important effect modifiers for cervical cancer risk [26].

Fig. 4.5.5: *Rate Ratio (RR)* for cervical cancer among Swedish-born women and foreign-born women by age at migration (a), duration of residence (b) and country of birth [14]*

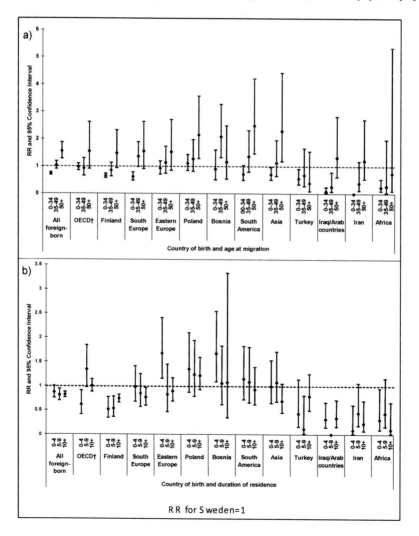

Montgomery and colleagues as well as Ekbom and colleagues investigated the risk of testicular cancer among Finnish immigrants to Sweden [27-28]. The latter study focused on the effect of age at immigration and duration of residence. Both studies were affected by lacking power and conclusions. In the most recent study by Beiki and colleagues on testicular cancer with high enough power, researchers found the risk of seminomas was statistical significantly modified by age at immigration and duration of residence among immigrants born in high-risk areas such as Denmark, Germany and Norway [16].

The effect of age at immigration and duration of residence was also part of the study on prostate cancer by Beiki and colleagues [15]. The risk of prostate cancer among immigrants was modified by duration of residence. However, the overall risk of prostate cancer was lower among immigrants compared to Swedish-born men in both strata of duration of residence (<40 and ≥40 years) or age at immigration (<35 and ≥35 years). This might suggest that either genetic factor are more influential than environmental factors in the susceptibility to prostate cancer, or more likely that it takes more than one generation for environmental factors to act.

Studies on cancer in Sweden-born individuals with foreign-born parents

In the study on testicular cancer among Sweden-born individuals with foreign foreign-born parents in Sweden by Beiki and colleagues [16], a statistically significant convergence of testicular cancer risk towards the risk of natives Swedes was observed. Furthermore, no significant difference across parental categories of origin (mother foreign-born, father foreign-born or both foreign-born) was found. However, Sweden-born men with both parents born in high-risk areas outside Sweden had an about 50% higher testicular cancer risk compared with Sweden-born men with both parents born in Sweden. While Sweden-born men with parents born in low-risk areas had about 15% lower risk compared with Sweden-born men with both parents born in Sweden.

Hemminki and colleagues analysed the risk of nervous system tumours, leukaemia and non-Hodgkin's lymphoma among Sweden-born children of immigrants [22]. An excess in the risk of non-Hodgkin's lymphoma was found among the offspring of Yugoslavian fathers and Turkish parents. In another study on Sweden-born children of immigrants, decreased risks were observed for breast cancer among Norwegian descendants, melanoma among descendants of Hungarian fathers and ovarian and bladder cancer among descendents of Finnish mothers, all consistent with the difference in cancer incidence between Swedes and the indigenous populations [20].

Cancer survival and mortality among immigrants

In a study on migrant population, cancer survival among Estonian immigrants in Sweden was compared to the total population of Sweden and to Estonians living in Estonia [29]. The survival rates of Estonians living in Sweden and the total population of Sweden were higher than that of the Estonians living in Estonia. Differences in survival between these population groups were found for cancers of the prostate, colon, lung, breast and ovary. It was concluded that most differences in cancer survival between Estonia and Sweden might be due to differences in socio-economic development.

Researchers at the Karolinska Institutet also performed a study to compare female breast cancer mortality among first- and second-generation immigrants with those among Swedish-born women [5]. For this purpose, a nation-wide cohort of 4.6 million women was followed between 1961 and 2007. A significantly higher all-cause mortality in some immigrant groups and their offspring was found in comparison with Sweden-born women with parents born in Sweden. However, the overall all-cause and breast cancer mortality was similar between immigrants and their offspring born in Sweden and Sweden-born women with Sweden-born parents. Cause-specific mortality increased significantly by increasing age at immigration and was statistically significantly higher among first-generation immigrants if breast cancer was diagnosed post-menopausally or in most recent years (years 2001-2007). Fifty percent higher breast cancer mortality was found among women with lowest versus highest educational level regardless of migration status (immigrants and their offspring, Sweden-born with Sweden-born parents).

4.5.5 Possibilities to combine cancer cases and denominator population

Sweden possesses unique health registries, providing great potentials to conduct register-based research in the area of migrant studies. The personal identity number (PIN) represents a key instrument, facilitating the conduct of migration-sensitive studies on cancer risk in Sweden. Country of birth, a currently most accepted proxy for ethnicity, is available in the Swedish Population Register and linkage to different demographic and health registers is easily possible.

By linking population registers and multi-generation registers to cancer and death registers, researchers are able to perform comparisons on incidence, mortality and survival for all types of cancer between immigrants, their descendents and native Swedes. In such studies, the denominator can be extracted from the Swedish Population Register and the numerator will be derived from cancer and death registers. It is also possible to retrieve other covariables such as socio-economic position (SEP) from demographic registers such as censuses and The Longitudinal Integration Database for Health Insurance and Labour Market studies. For example, researchers from the Karolinska Institutet in studies performed on cervical, endometrial, ovarian, breast and prostate cancers were able to adjust calculated relative risks by SEP [5, 14-15].

Through the national health care quality registers it is also possible to acquire more clinical data for specific cancer types. We are currently conducting studies on cancer risks in immigrants focusing on treatments, access to health care and cancer stages.

One problem with regard to performing migrant studies in Sweden is the lack of information on ethnicity. Different ethnic groups may have dissimilarities in factors (i.e. life style, genetic, socioeconomic, and educational background, health status and language proficiency) affecting the health outcomes and yet born in the same country. Thus, taking ethnicity into consideration will help to clarify findings of migrant studies.

The long standing use of registers in Sweden provides sufficient evidence that their use is safe regarding protection of the individual's right to non-disclosure of the data.

Further future actions can be:

- Improving the quality and expanding the content of data on migrant populations in the registers;
- Facilitating access to data from registers using new technical solutions, such as federated but physically distributed databases;
- Focusing on other aspects of cancer research such as survival, mortality and access to health care and type of treatment.

References

1. Swedish Tax Agency. Population registration in Sweden. 2007 [cited 2010 January 20]; Edition 4:[Available from: http://www.skatteverket.se/download/18.5cbdbba811c9a 768f0c80002830/717b04.pdf?posid=1&sv.search.query.allwords=717b04.pdf.
2. Ludvigsson, J.F., et al., The Swedish personal identity number: possibilities and pitfalls in healthcare and medical research. Eur J Epidemiol, 2009. 24(11): p. 659-67.
3. Wikipedia. Sweden. 2010; Available from: http://en.wikipedia.org/wiki/Sweden.
4. Statistics Sweden. 2010 [cited 2010 January 20]; Available from: www.scb.se.
5. Beiki, o., Cancer and migration: Epidemiological studies on relationship between country of birth, socio-economic position and cancer. 2010, Karolinska Institutet: Stockholm.
6. Official Statistics of Sweden, Census of the Population and Housing in 1960: Report on the planning and processing of the Census of the Population and Housing. 1965, Stockholm, Sweden: Statistics Sweden.
7. Official Statistics of Sweden, Census of the Population and Housing in 1970, part 13: Occupation and education. 1975, Stockholm, Sweden: Statistics Sweden.
8. Statistics Sweden. 2002. Reports on Statistical Co-ordination for the Official Statistics of Sweden 2002:3. Statistics on persons with foreign background. Guidelines and recommendations.

9. Barlow, L., et al., The completeness of the Swedish Cancer Register: a sample survey for year 1998. Acta Oncol, 2009. 48(1): p. 27-33.

10. Holmang, S., et al., Completeness and correctness of registration of renal pelvic and ureteral cancer in the Swedish Cancer Registry. Scand J Urol Nephrol, 2008. 42(1): p. 12-7.

11. Turesson, I., et al., Ascertainment and diagnostic accuracy for hematopoietic lymphoproliferative malignancies in Sweden 1964-2003. Int J Cancer, 2007. 121(10): p. 2260-6.

12. Mattsson, B. and A. Wallgren, Completeness of the Swedish Cancer Register. Nonnotified cancer cases recorded on death certificates in 1978. Acta Radiol Oncol, 1984. 23(5): p. 305-13.

13. Swedish Association of Local Authorities and Regions (SALAR), National Health Care Quality Registries in Sweden. 2007: Stockholm.

14. Beiki, O., et al., Cervical, endometrial and ovarian cancers among immigrants in Sweden: importance of age at migration and duration of residence. Eur J Cancer, 2009. 45(1): p. 107-18.

15. Beiki, O., et al., Risk of prostate cancer among Swedish-born and foreign-born men in Sweden, 1961-2004. Int J Cancer, 2009. 124(8): p. 1941-53.

16. Beiki, O., et al., Subtype-specific risk of testicular tumors among immigrants and their descendants in Sweden, 1960 to 2007. Cancer Epidemiol Biomarkers Prev, 2010. 19(4): p. 1053-65.

17. Moradi, T., et al., Risk of thyroid cancer among Iranian immigrants in Sweden. Cancer Causes Control, 2008. 19(3): p. 221-6.

18. Hemminki, K., et al., The Swedish Family-Cancer Database 2009: prospects for histology-specific and immigrant studies. Int J Cancer, 2009.

19. Eggert, J. and K. Sundquist, Socioeconomic factors, country of birth, and years in Sweden are associated with first birth fertility trends during the 1990s: a national cohort study. Scand J Public Health, 2006. 34(5): p. 504-14.

20. Hemminki, K. and X. Li, Cancer risks in second-generation immigrants to Sweden. Int J Cancer, 2002. 99(2): p. 229-37.

21. Hemminki, K. and X. Li, Cancer risks in childhood and adolescence among the offspring of immigrants to Sweden. Br J Cancer, 2002. 86(9): p. 1414-8.

22. Hemminki, K., X. Li, and K. Czene, Cancer risks in first-generation immigrants to Sweden. Int J Cancer, 2002. 99(2): p. 218-28.

23. Mousavi, S.M., et al., Cancer incidence among Iranian immigrants in Sweden and Iranian residents compared to the native Swedish population. Eur J Cancer, 2009.

24. Nilsson, B., et al., Cancer incidence in Estonian migrants to Sweden. Int J Cancer, 1993. 55(2): p. 190-5.

25. Zendehdel, K., et al., Cancer Incidence Rates among Iranian immigrants in Sweden, a Retrospective Population-Based Cohort Study (Manuscript).

26. Azerkan, F., et al., Risk of cervical cancer among immigrants by age at immigration and follow-up time in Sweden, from 1968 to 2004. Int J Cancer, 2008. 123(11): p. 2664-70.

27. Ekbom, A., et al., Age at immigration and duration of stay in relation to risk for testicular cancer among Finnish immigrants in Sweden. J Natl Cancer Inst, 2003. 95(16): p. 1238-40.

28. Montgomery, S.M., et al., Germ-cell testicular cancer in offspring of Finnish immigrants to Sweden. Cancer Epidemiol Biomarkers Prev, 2005. 14(1): p. 280-2.

29. Nilsson, B., et al., Cancer survival in Estonian migrants to Sweden. J Epidemiol Community Health, 1997. 51(4): p. 418-23.

Chapter 5:

Conclusion

5. Conclusion

Melina Arnold[1], Oliver Razum[1], Anna Reeske[2], Jacob Spallek[1,2]

1   Bielefeld University, Department for Epidemiology and International Public Health, Germany
2   University of Bremen, Bremen Institute for Prevention Research and Social Medicine, Germany

Rapidly increasing ethnic diversity of European societies entails the transition and new orientation of social systems, especially concerning the maintenance of adequate, purposeful and high quality healthcare. Migration-sensitive monitoring of health is essential in order to assess and react to changing health care needs of culturally diverse groups and thus also of European societies as a whole. This work for the first time presents a detailed overview and methodological discussion of migration-sensitive cancer registration in selected European countries.

Aim of this book was to describe the status quo of migrant-sensitive cancer registration in Europe and reveal and discuss the potentials regarding a routine monitoring of the health and cancer patterns among migrant populations in Europe. This was achieved by presenting case reports from five European country, arisen from close collaborations with local experts. These reports enable a more profound view on country-specific potentials and barriers of migration-sensitive cancer registration and research in Europe as a whole. The key facts from all country reports are outlined in table 5.1.

Country-specific insights

Germany, The Netherlands and Sweden are typical immigration countries with more than 10% of the entire population having some kind of migration background and a large fraction of migrant from non-Western countries such as Turkey, Morocco, the Caribbean, Eastern Europe, the Middle East. Given those facts, one should actually assume some degree of adaptation of (health) data acquisition procedures to a changing composition of societies with changing needs and expectations. In cancer registration, The Netherlands and Sweden have adapted most with regard to the relevance and importance of migration-sensitive data collection, being evident in sophisticated data gathering, linkage and targeted utilization for scientific purposes. This requires highly developed technical solutions and funds allowing for the inclusion of migration-sensitive variables in the course of routine analyses as well as the handling of directed research questions. However, lacking or incomplete information on ethnicity, especially in respect of the limitations accompanied by the use of country of birth as identification method for migrants, still appears to be a barrier. Both Sweden and The

Tab. 5.1:   *Migration-sensitive cancer registration in selected European countries –*
potentials and barriers

Country	Migrants in general population, (2) Largest migrant groups (origin)*	Indicators available in (1) Population data, (2) Cancer registry data
Finland: Finnish Cancer Registry *(population-based, national level)*	(1) 4.4% (foreign country of birth) (2) Russia, Estonia	(1) Country of birth, Citizenship, Language (2) None
Germany: Regional registries *(all 16 federal states covered in 2011, completeness fits international standards in 14 federal states)*	(1) ~20% (migration background) (2) Eastern Europe (resettlers), South and South Eastern Europe (Turkey)	(1) None (Country of birth in Mikrocensus data) (2) None.
Netherlands: Netherlands Cancer Registry *(population-based, national level)*	(1) 19.5% (foreign background) (2) Turkey, Morocco, Western Europe, Suriname, Netherlands Antilles, Indonesia	(1) Country of birth (2) Country of birth
Scotland: Scottish Cancer Registry *(population-based, national level)*	(1) 3.8% (foreign country of birth) (2) UK, US, Western Europe, Pakistan, India, Bangladesh, China	(1) Ethnic group (category classification, predefined in Scottish census) (2) Ethnic group (classification varies)
Sweden: Swedish Cancer Register *(population-based, national level)*	(1) 13.8% (foreign country of birth) (2) Europe (mostly Scandinavia), Iraq, Iran, Former Yugoslavia, Poland	(1) Country of birth, foreign background (2) None.

*   latest data available
CHI = Community Health Index; CR = Cancer Registry/Registration; CSN = Citizen Service Number;
FSU = Former Soviet Union; PID/PIN = Personal Identity/ Identification Number

Tab. 5.1 (continued)

Routine analyses? Studies on cancer in migrants (key references)	Main barriers	Current/Future Potentials
• No. • Using linkage procedures [22]	• Time consuming permission procedures • Costs of additional data extraction • Small number of cancer cases among migrants	• Data linkage through personal identity code PID • Inclusion of country of origin in CR data
• No. • Using a name-based approach to identify Turkish cancer cases [1-3] • Setting up a historical cohort of resettlers from the FSU [4-5]	• Data protection not officially clarified • German history (prosecution of ethnic minorities) • Organisation of CRs on federal state level by federal state law → lacking data comparability • Lacking of migrant indicators in population data	• Indirect methods (e.g. name-based approaches) • Numerator-only analyses • Data linkage procedures
• No. • Using linkage procedures [6-8]	• No resources for routine analyses • Lacking completeness of country of birth variable in incidence analyses	• Introduction of citizen service number (CSN) will facilitate linkage
• No. • Using name-based approaches for migrants from India, Pakistan and China [9-11] • First attempts using linkage with CHI [12-13]	• Existing data often incomplete • Inconsistent coding of ethnic groups between data sources • Only small ethnic minority groups	• Linkage procedures using CHI are promising and can in future overcome most barriers
• Yes. • Using the Health and Migration Cohort [14-16] • Using the Family-Cancer Database [17-21]	• Lack of information on ethnicity (variation within the same country of origin) • Technical solutions are still under development	• PIN facilitates linkage of registers and enables all kinds of analyses (incidence, mortality, survival) and covariates (e.g. SES)

Netherlands introduced unique personal identification numbers in their health care systems, in order to facilitate networking and linkage. This procedure promises further analysis options in future and would also lead to a high degree of completeness in data. Due to a region-based cancer registration (at the cost of lacking data comparability between the federal states) and no migrant identification options in official longitudinal population or health data in Germany, research on cancer in migrants is only possible in very limited and laborious ways, e.g. by means of name-based approaches or historical cohorts. In addition, often insufficiently clarified data protection regulations prevail.

In Finland, migrants represent only a small fraction of the population and mainly originate from Russia and Estonia. Although country of birth, citizenship and spoken language are included in population data, the cancer registry does not routinely collect those variables. The assumed small number of cancer cases at a rather high expenditure of costs and time, does not seem to counterbalance the value that could be achieved with introducing such research and for instance the inclusion of country of birth in cancer registry data. However, also data linkage procedures using the personal identity code (PID), automatically assigned to every Finnish citizen, promise further options for conducting migration-sensitive cancer (and health) research in future.

Scotland also only hosts a relatively small number of migrants most often coming from Western countries as well as South Asian origins. The Scottish population census is being conducted on a decadal basis and includes a categorization of ethnic group. Scottish cancer registry data principally also include ethnic group, whereas the exact distinction of groups may vary between cancer and population data due to inconsistent coding. To overcome those difficulties, an attempt has been made using the personal identification number (PIN), facilitating linkage procedures and making all kinds of migration-sensitive analyses possible.

Migration-sensitive cancer registration: Main challenges

One of the major challenges in the conduct of migration-sensitive cancer research is the **definition and identification** of migrant groups as migrant background or ethnicity is a social construct that is hard to grasp. The understanding of "migrants" or "ethnic minority groups" can however vary strongly between countries, in each case associated to the history, dimension and cognition of migration in research and public respectively. This makes it difficult to develop and implement a uniform definition for all European countries. Furthermore, ethnologic and epidemiologic views on the concept "migration" or "culture" can deviate from each other in a sense that in most instances the chosen definition to identify migrants in population-based migration research is based on variables in routine health data that already exist, rather than on the most comprehensive concept for migrant status. The latter often require disproportional effort (new data gathering, setup of studies) while being very specific with regard to characteristics of certain migrant groups in the (restricted) catchment area of the cancer registry respectively and are thus often not applicable using routine data. At present, the most accepted concept for identification of migrants is country of birth, when applicable refined with more profound/detailed variables such as religion or spoken language, allowing for clear demarcations on the one hand, but lacking the possibility to make distinctions regarding ethnic diversity within migrant groups and to identify the offspring of migrants.

A further challenge is the development and implementation of migration-sensitive health (cancer) indicators. They can be seen as a valuable method to provide important insights into existing cancer disparities just like into differences in underlying risk factor patterns and possible starting points for public health and prevention strategies. Yet, as we also found in our survey, routine data sources and cancer registries may not include a person's ethnicity or country of birth at all. When direct methods to perform migration-sensitive analyses (migrants are equally identified in both numerator – cancer registry data – and denominator – the reference population –) are hence not possible, indirect methods (based on linkage procedures) can serve as good alternatives although they involve quite some technical effort and may be impeded in connection with data privacy regulations that demand strict adherence. Linkage procedures require a proxy of ethnicity in any population-based data source (e.g. population census data or data from statistical offices) and can be applied either based on probability matching or personalized identifiers used in some countries.

Migrant studies are often subject to specific **biases** that should always be taken into account when conducting research in this field. Most prominent are biases with regard to selection effects ("healthy migrant effect", "salmon bias"), identification methods (as discussed above) and confounding effects (especially the effects of socioeconomic circumstances and their interaction with migrant status). Furthermore, differences in data quality between countries (e.g. disparities in the coding of causes of death, availability/implementation of cancer screening and diagnostic procedures) can lead to considerable bias.

Recommendations for the next steps towards a migration-sensitive cancer registration

In this work, we identified barriers as well as potentials of migration-sensitive cancer registration in Europe. We demonstrated the challenges related to migration-sensitive cancer registration when it comes to the identification of migrants, the integration of migration-sensitive components into existing health indicators as well as the conduct of analyses with possible threats to validity due to biases that may emerge and need to be kept in mind. Furthermore, ways to overcome those difficulties by selecting alternative approaches or making use of (new) linkage options were presented and have already exemplarily been implemented in some European countries.

In summary, migration-sensitive cancer registration and monitoring is at different stages in different European countries. Its implementation is highly dependent on the (i) national context, (ii) the relevance of migrant groups within a country, (iii) the availability of corresponding resources as well as (iv) the backup from politics. Most importantly and in view of an increasing culturally diverse European society, the necessity for migration-sensitive cancer registration first of all deserves awareness on various levels. Existing heterogeneities in data infrastructure between and within countries require some overlap, i.e. a minimal set of consistent definitions and indicators in order to ensure a certain degree of data comparability.

Until the implementation of routine monitoring, a essential prerequisite is to perform additional research and analytical studies in terms of within and cross-country analyses to study the feasibility and problems of migrations-sensitive cancer registration across Europe. Furthermore, results from such research can help gain further insight into explanations for different cancer patterns and give rise to directed prevention strategies in ethnic minority groups. On this account, migration-sensitive health research needs to be vitalized and augmented by intensive networking between (and sometimes firstly even within) countries in future.

References

1. Spallek, J., et al., Cancer incidence rate ratios of Turkish immigrants in Hamburg, Germany: A registry based study. Cancer epidemiology, 2009. 33(6): p. 413-8.
2. Zeeb, H., et al., Transition in cancer patterns among Turks residing in Germany. Eur J Cancer, 2002. 38(5): p. 705-11.
3. Spallek, J., et al., Cancer patterns among children of Turkish descent in Germany: a study at the German Childhood Cancer Registry. BMC Public Health, 2008. 8: p. 152.
4. Kyobutungi, C., et al., Mortality from cancer among ethnic German immigrants from the Former Soviet Union, in Germany. Eur J Cancer, 2006. 42(15): p. 2577-84.
5. Ronellenfitsch, U., et al., Stomach cancer mortality in two large cohorts of migrants from the Former Soviet Union to Israel and Germany: are there implications for prevention? Eur J Gastroenterol Hepatol, 2009. 21(4): p. 409-16.
6. Stirbu, I., et al., Cancer mortality rates among first and second generation migrants in the Netherlands: Convergence toward the rates of the native Dutch population. Int J Cancer, 2006. 119(11): p. 2665-72.
7. Bos, V., et al., Ethnic inequalities in age- and cause-specific mortality in The Netherlands. Int J Epidemiol, 2004. 33(5): p. 1112-9.

8. Visser, O. and F.E. van Leeuwen, Cancer risk in first generation migrants in North-Holland/Flevoland, The Netherlands, 1995-2004. Eur J Cancer, 2007. 43(5): p. 901-8.

9. Merchant, N.E., et al., Oral carcinoma in the Indian and Pakistani community in Scotland. J Oral Med, 1986. 41(1): p. 62-5.

10. Matheson, L.M., et al., Incidence of colo-rectal, breast and lung cancer in a Scottish Asian population. Health Bull (Edinb), 1985. 43(5): p. 245-9.

11. Muir, C.S., Epidemiology of cancer in ethnic groups. Br J Cancer Suppl, 1996. 29: p. S12-6.

12. Bhopal, R., et al., Cohort profile: Scottish Health and Ethnicity Linkage Study of 4.65 million people exploring ethnic variations in disease in Scotland. Int J Epidemiol, 2010.

13. Fischbacher, C.M., et al., Record linked retrospective cohort study of 4.6 million people exploring ethnic variations in disease: myocardial infarction in South Asians. BMC Public Health, 2007. 7: p. 142.

14. Beiki, O., et al., Risk of prostate cancer among Swedish-born and foreign-born men in Sweden, 1961-2004. International Journal of Cancer, 2009. 124(8): p. 1941-1953.

15. Moradi, T., et al., Risk of thyroid cancer among Iranian immigrants in Sweden. Cancer Causes Control, 2008. 19(3): p. 221-6.

16. Beiki, O., et al., Subtype-Specific Risk of Testicular Tumors among Immigrants and Their Descendants in Sweden, 1960 to 2007. Cancer Epidemiology Biomarkers & Prevention, 2010. 19(4): p. 1053-1065.

17. Eggert, J. and K. Sundquist, Socioeconomic factors, country of birth, and years in Sweden are associated with first birth fertility trends during the 1990s: A national cohort study. Scandinavian Journal of Public Health, 2006. 34(5): p. 504-514.

18. Mousavi, S.M., et al., Cancer incidence among Iranian immigrants in Sweden and Iranian residents compared to the native Swedish population. European Journal of Cancer, 2010. 46(3): p. 599-605.

19. Hemminki, K., X. Li, and K. Czene, Cancer risks in first-generation immigrants to Sweden. Int J Cancer, 2002. 99(2): p. 218-28.

20. Hemminki, K. and X. Li, Cancer risks in second-generation immigrants to Sweden. Int J Cancer, 2002. 99(2): p. 229-37.

21. Hemminki, K., et al., The Swedish Family-Cancer Database 2009: prospects for histology-specific and immigrant studies. International Journal of Cancer, 2010. 126(10): p. 2259-2267.

22. Soininen, L., S. Jarvinen, and E. Pukkala, Cancer incidence among Sami in Northern Finland, 1979-1998. Int J Cancer, 2002. 100(3): p. 342-6.

Challenges in Public Health

Im Zeitalter der Globalisierung lässt sich *Public Health* nicht mehr allein innerhalb von nationalen Grenzen betreiben: Pandemien, abnehmende Trinkwasservorräte und steigender Tabakkonsum sind nur einige Beispiele für eine Vielzahl von neuen Herausforderungen, die einen weiter reichenden, internationalen Blick erfordern. Zusätzlich trägt eine einseitig an Wirtschaftsinteressen orientierte Globalisierung zu der weltweit zunehmenden gesundheitlichen Ungleichheit bei. Die Globalisierung eröffnet andererseits aber neue Wege, auch über Staatsgrenzen und große Entfernungen hinweg Wissen und Erfahrungen auszutauschen und gemeinschaftlich zu handeln. Kernpunkte für *Public Health* sind dabei die international vergleichende Analyse von Gesundheitsproblemen und möglichen Lösungsansätzen sowie die wissenschaftlich basierte und gerechte Ausgestaltung von Gesundheitssystemen. Hierzu möchte die Buchreihe *Challenges in Public Health* einen Beitrag leisten.

In times of globalisation, Public Health can no longer be practiced within national borders alone. Pandemics, diminishing drinking water supplies and increasing tobacco consumption are examples of the many new challenges that require a cross-border, international approach. In addition, a globalisation that is narrowly focused on economic interests contributes to growing health inequalities worldwide. At the same time, globalisation offers new opportunities to exchange knowledge and experiences and to collaborate across national borders. Key issues for Public Health are an international comparison of health problems and of possible strategies to solve them, as well as an evidence-based and equitable development of health systems. The book series *Challenges in Public Health* aims to contribute to this endeavour.

Band 18 Gerhard Heller: Krankheitskonzepte und Krankheitssymptome. Eine empirische Untersuchung bei den Tamang von Cautara/Nepal zur Frage der kulturspezifischen Prägung von Krankheitserleben. 1985.

Band 19 Hans-Jochen Diesfeld / Sigrid Wolter (Hrsg.): Medizin in Entwicklungsländern. Handbuch zur praxisorientierten Vorbereitung für medizinische Entwicklungshelfer. 5. neubearbeitete Auflage. 1989.

Band 20 Verena Kücholl: Soziokulturelle Wege des Heilens. Eine ethnomedizinische Analyse und Interpretation des Samkhya und der Heiltradition der Navajo. 1985.

Band 21 Frank-Peter Schelp (Ed.): Health Problems in Asia and in the Federal Republic of Germany. How to solve them? Proceedings of a seminar on "Techniques and Problems of Intervention Trials in Developing and Developed Countries". 1985.

Band 22 Rolf Heinmüller, Winfried Kern: Primäre Gesundheitsversorgung im südwestlichen Sudan. Eine Feldforschung bei den südsudanesischen Azande zur Evaluierung der Einflüsse des 'Primary Health Care'-Programms auf gesundheitliche Lage und allgemeine Lebensbedingungen. Detailed English Summary. 1987.

Band 23 Andreas Hahold/Axel Kroeger: Krankheitsbewältigung im Andenhochland Perus. Ergebnisse einer Bevölkerungsbefragung. 1986.

Band 24 Georg Kamm / Peter Witton / Hatibu Lweno: Anaesthesia Notebook for Medical Auxilaries. With special Reference to Anaesthesia Practice in Developing Countries. 1989.

Band 25 Alice S. Kuhn: Heiler und ihre Patienten auf dem Dach der Welt. Ladakh aus ethnomedizinischer Sicht. 1988.

Band 26 Wolfgang Bichmann: Community Involvement in Nepal's Health System. A case study of district health services management and the Community Health Leader scheme in Kaski district. 1989.

Band 27 M. Luisa Vázquez / Renate Lipowsky / Axel Kroeger: Malaria und kutane Leishmaniase in Kolumbien. Vorkommen, Volkskonzepte und traditionelle Behandlungsformen. 1989.

Band 28 Heinrich Berg / Axel Kroeger / Carmen Perez-Samaniego / Fernando Malo: Kranke Menschen – krankes Gesundheitswesen? Eine epidemiologische Untersuchung in Nord-Mexiko. 1989.

Band 29 Emmie Ho-Tsui / Margit Urhahn: Medizin und Gesundheitsforschung in Entwicklungsländern. Bibliographie des Instituts für Tropenhygiene 1984-1988. 1991.

Band 30 Thomas Lux: Gespräche mit afrikanischen Krankenpflegern und Heilern. Bilder von Krankheit im Mikrokosmos von Malanville(Benin), 1991.

Band 31 Christopher Knauth: Arzneimittelgebrauch armer Bevölkerungsschichten in städtischen Elendsvierteln Perus. Möglichkeiten und Grenzen der Gesundheitserziehung zum rationalen Arzneimittelgebrauch. 1991.

Band 32 Erhard Hinz: Geomedizinische und biogeographische Aspekte der Krankheitsverbreitung und Gesundheitsversorgung in Industrie- und Entwicklungsländern. 1991.

Band 33 Klaus Hoffmann: Psychiatrie in Afrika. Eine Einführung für Entwicklungshelfer. 1992.

Band 34 Dorothea Sich / Hans Jochen Diesfeld / Angelika Deigner / Monika Habermann (Hrsg.): Medizin und Kultur. Eine Propädeutik für Studierende der Medizin und der Ethnologie mit 4 Seminaren in Kulturvergleichender Medizinischer Anthropologie (KMA). 1993. 2., unveränd. Aufl. 1995.

Band 35 Annette Wiemann-Michaels: Die verhexte Speise. Eine ethnopsychosomatische Studie über das Depressive Syndrom in Nepal. 1994.

Band 36 Christine Loytved: Hebammen in Ozeanien zwischen traditioneller und westlicher Medizin. Weiterbildung traditioneller Hebammen in Westsamoa und Tonga. 1994.

Band 37 Andrea Materlik: Medizinisch-anthropologische Aspekte von Lepra im Amazonas und ihre Bedeutung für die Gesundheitserziehung. 1994.

Band 38 Oliver Razum: Improving Service Quality through Action Research, as applied in the Expanded Programme on Immunization (EPI). 1994.

Band 39 Ulrich Schramm: Einflußfaktoren auf die Akzeptanz von baulichen Anlagen der ländlichen Gesundheitseinheiten in Ägypten. Fallstudie am Beispiel der staatlichen Einheit in Zebeda unter Verwendung der Post-Occupancy Evaluation. 1995.

Band 40 Rainer Sauerborn / Adrien Nougtara / Hans Jochen Diesfeld (Eds.): Recherche sur les systèmes de santé: Le cas de la zone médicale de Solenzo, Burkina Faso. Auteurs: Rainer Sauerborn, Adrien Nougtara, Hans Jochen Diesfeld, Gaston Sorgho, Joseph Bidiga, Lougousse Tiébélessé, Eric Latimer, Roberto Sallier de La Tour, Uwe Brinkmann, Don Shepard. 1995.

Band 41 Rainer Sauerborn / Adrien Nougtara / Hans Jochen Diesfeld (Eds.): Les Côuts Economiques de la Maladie pour les Ménages au Milieu Rural du Burkina Faso. Avec des contributions de Rainer Sauerborn, Adrien Nougtara, Maurice Hien, Issouf Ibrango, Matthias Borchert, Justus Benzler, Eberhard Koob, Hans Jochen Diesfeld. 1996.

Band 42 Erhard Hinz: Helminthiasen des Menschen in Thailand. 1996.

Band 43 Matthias Perleth: Historical Aspects of American Trypanosomiasis (Chagas' Disease). 1997.

Band 44 Christiane Fischer: Über die Effektivität der Dorfgesundheitsarbeiterinnen innerhalb der Nichtregierungsorganisation ACCORD in Tamil Nadu/Südindien. Aktionsforschung im Rahmen der Gesundheitssystemforschung. 1998.

Band 45 Maureen Dar Iang: Assessment of antenatal and obstetric care services in a rural district of Nepal. 1999.

Band 46 Julia Katzan: sòi mendan – Die Sache mit dem Wasser... Eine medizinethnologische Untersuchung zum Zusammenhang von Wasser und Krankheit aus indigener Sicht. 2001.

Band 47 Catharina Will: Malaria-Selbstmedikation mit Chloroquin in einem hyperendemischen Gebiet (Mali). 2001.

Band 48 Ansgar Gerhardus: Entscheidungsprozesse im Gesundheitssektor. Der Beitrag der Theorie der politischen Ökonomie. 2001.

Band 49 Sylvie Schuster: Der Schwangerschaftsabbruch im Grasland Kameruns. Medizin, Kultur und Praxis. 2004.

Band 50 Sascha Klotzbücher: Das ländliche Gesundheitswesen der VR China. Strukturen – Akteure – Dynamik. 2006.

Challenges in Public Health

Editor: Prof. Dr. Oliver Razum

Band 51 Ulrich Ronellenfitsch: Cardiovascular Mortality among Ethnic German Immigrants from the Former Soviet Union. 2007.

Band 52 Manuela De Allegri: To Enrol or not to Enrol in Community Health Insurance. Case Study from Burkina Faso. 2007.

Band 53 Catherine Kyobutungi: Ethnic German Immigrants from the Former Soviet Union: Mortality from External Causes and Cancers. 2008.

www.peterlang.de